ABC of
Emergency Differential Diagnosis

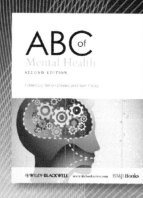
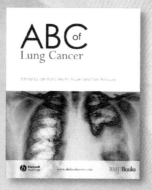
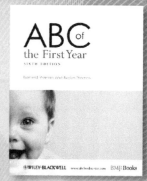
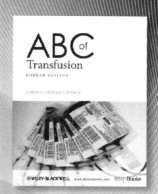
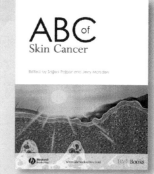
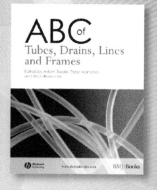

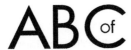

ABC of

Emergency Differential Diagnosis

EDITED BY

Francis Morris
Consultant in Emergency Medicine
Emergency Department
Northern General Hospital
Sheffield, UK

Alan Fletcher
Consultant in Acute Medicine and Emergency Medicine
Emergency Department
Northern General Hospital
Sheffield, UK

WILEY-BLACKWELL

A John Wiley & Sons, Ltd., Publication

BMJ｜Books

This edition first published 2009, © 2009 by Blackwell Publishing Ltd

BMJ Books is an imprint of BMJ Publishing Group Limited, used under licence by Blackwell Publishing which was acquired by John Wiley & Sons in February 2007. Blackwell's publishing programme has been merged with Wiley's global Scientific, Technical and Medical business to form Wiley-Blackwell.

Registered office: John Wiley & Sons Ltd, The Atrium, Southern Gate, Chichester, West Sussex, PO19 8SQ, UK

Editorial offices: 9600 Garsington Road, Oxford, OX4 2DQ, UK
The Atrium, Southern Gate, Chichester, West Sussex, PO19 8SQ, UK
111 River Street, Hoboken, NJ 07030-5774, USA

For details of our global editorial offices, for customer services and for information about how to apply for permission to reuse the copyright material in this book please see our website at www.wiley.com/wiley-blackwell

Library of Congress Cataloging-in-Publication Data
ABC of emergency differential diagnosis / edited by Francis Morris, Alan Fletcher.
      p. ; cm.
   Includes bibliographical references and index.
   ISBN 978-1-4051-7063-5
      1. Diagnosis, Differential--Case studies. 2. Medical emergencies--Diagnosis--Case studies. I. Morris, Francis.
II. Fletcher, Alan, 1968- III. Title: Emergency differential diagnosis.
   [DNLM: 1. Diagnosis, Differential--Case Reports. 2. Emergency Treatment--Case Reports. WB 141.5 A137 2009]
   RC71.5.A23 2009
   616.07'5--dc22

                                                                             2009004444

ISBN: 978-1-4051-7063-5

A catalogue record for this book is available from the British Library.

Set in 9.25/12 pt Minion by Newgen Imaging Systems (P) Ltd, Chennai, India
Printed & bound in Singapore

Contents

Contributors

Arun Chaudhuri

Consultant Acute Physician, Ninewells Hospital and Medical School, Dundee, UK

Sue Croft

SpR in Emergency Medicine and Acute Medicine, Medical Assessment Unit, Northern General Hospital, Sheffield, UK

Roger Dalton

SpR in Emergency Medicine, Emergency Department, Northern General Hospital, Sheffield, UK

Scott Davison

General Practitioner, Crystal Peaks Medical Centre, Peaks Mount, Sheffield, UK

Nicki Doddridge

Consultant in Acute Medicine, Emergency Department, Northern General Hospital, Sheffield, UK

Duncan Drury

SpR in General Surgery, Sheffield Teaching Hospitals NHS Foundation Trust, Sheffield, UK

Alan Fletcher

Consultant in Acute Medicine and Emergency Medicine, Emergency Department, Northern General Hospital, Sheffield, UK

Rachel Foster

SpR in Infectious Diseases, Royal Hallamshire Hospital, Sheffield, UK

Claire Gardner

SpR in Acute Medicine, Emergency Department, Northern General Hospital, Sheffield, UK

Carole Gavin

Consultant in Emergency Medicine, Salford Hospital, Salford, UK

Steve Goodacre

Professor in Emergency Medicine, Emergency Department, Northern General Hospital, Sheffield, UK

Charles Heatley

General Practitioner, Birley Health Centre, Sheffield, UK

Sian Ireland

Consultant in Emergency Medicine, Royal Cornwall Hospital, Truro, Cornwall, UK

Kevin Jones

Consultant Physician, Acute Medical Receiving Unit, Royal Bolton Hospital, Bolton, UK

Richard Kendall

Consultant in Emergency Medicine, Addenbrookes Hospital, Cambridge, UK

Peter Lawson

Consultant Physician and Geriatrician, Northern General Hospital, Sheffield, UK

Tom Locker

Consultant in Emergency Medicine, Barnsley District General Hospital, Barnsley, UK

Suzanne Mason

Reader in Emergency Medicine, Northern General Hospital, Sheffield, UK

Francis Morris

Consultant in Emergency Medicine, Emergency Department, Northern General Hospital, Sheffield, UK

Alastair Pickering

Academic Clinical Lecturer and SpR in Emergency Medicine, Hull Royal Infirmary, Hull, UK

Karen Selby

Consultant in Obstetrics and Gynaecology, Jessop Hospital for Women, Sheffield, UK

Rachel Tattersall

Consultant Rheumatologist, Royal Hallamshire Hospital, Sheffield, UK

Preface

What makes a good doctor? One of many essential attributes is the ability to take a good history, appropriately examine, and apply sound clinical judgement to reach the correct diagnosis.

All 19 chapters in this book have the same format. Each starts with a patient's history concerning a common complaint and asks you, the reader, to generate a differential diagnosis based upon the information supplied. This is then followed by the examination findings, thus helping you refine the diagnostic process so that you are able to arrive at a single principal working diagnosis. The emergency management of this condition is then discussed.

Our hope is that working through these cases will be enjoyable, and that you will refine your diagnostic skills.

Francis Morris
Alan Fletcher

CHAPTER 1

Unconsciousness and Coma

Roger Dalton

CASE HISTORY

A 57-year-old man is found in an unconscious state at home. He was in bed when his wife left at 7.00 a.m. that morning to go to work. On her return home at 3.45 p.m., he was still in the same position in bed, unrousable, incontinent of urine, and the cup of tea she had left for him was untouched. He has been unwell recently, and prescribed a course of antibiotics and co-codamol from his General Practitioner for a discharging ear infection. He suffers from hypertension, type 2 diabetes mellitus and long-standing depression. His medication list shows that he has been prescribed gliclazide 80 mg twice daily, atenolol 25 mg once daily, ramipril 5 mg once daily and amitriptyline 25 mg once daily. He has no known allergies. His wife informs you that he has had bad headaches recently, but that no-one else at home has been unwell.

Question: What differential diagnosis would you consider from the history?

This man is in a coma, which is defined as 'unrousable unresponsiveness'. Using the objective clinical assessment tool, the Glasgow Coma Score (see Table 1.1), coma is defined as a score of 8 or less. Those patients with a score between 14 and 9 are defined as having altered consciousness and those with a top score of 15 are normal, alert and orientated. When considering a differential diagnosis for the cause of a patient's unresponsiveness it is important to consider those conditions that are easily reversible first.

Hypoglycaemia

The patient is a known diabetic. Hypoglycaemia or, less commonly, hyperglycaemia can result in altered consciousness and must be actively diagnosed and promptly treated. A simple bedside glucose test will identify abnormalities in blood glucose levels and will guide appropriate therapy.

It is essential that any patient with confusion, altered consciousness, coma or focal neurological signs has their blood glucose estimated as part of the initial assessment. Neurological signs resulting from hypoglycaemia usually resolve quickly with treatment, though

Table 1.1 The Glasgow Coma Score.

Eye opening	
Spontaneously	4
To speech	3
To pain	2
None	1
Verbal response	
Orientated	5
Disorientated speech	4
Inappropriate words	3
Incomprehensible sounds	2
None	1
Motor response	
Obeys commands	6
Localises painful stimuli	5
Withdrawal from pain	4
Flexion to pain	3
Extension to pain	2
None	1

Box 1.1 Drugs that can affect conscious level

- Alcohol
- Opiates
- Benzodiazepines
- Tricyclic antidepressants
- Street drugs, e.g. gamma-hydroxybutyric acid (GHB)

---

the failure to recognise and treat hypoglycaemia promptly may lead to permanent neurological damage.

Drugs and alcohol

Excess alcohol with or without other prescription or recreational drugs is the commonest cause of altered consciousness and not quickly reversible. Of all the drugs that affect a patient's consciousness (see Box 1.1) opiates are the only group that are readily treatable. Opiate excess leads to coma, and life-threatening respiratory depression, but thankfully can be quickly and effectively treated by the antagonist naloxone. The signs of opiate poisoning are seen in Box 1.2. Naloxone should be administered to any patient with any signs compatible with opiate poisoning.

ABC of Emergency Differential Diagnosis. Edited by F. Morris and A. Fletcher.
© 2009 Blackwell Publishing, ISBN: 978-1-4051-7063-5.

Box 1.2 **Signs of opiate ingestion**

- Depressed conscious level
- Depressed respiratory rate
- Pin point pupils
- Needlestick trackmarks

Box 1.3 **Signs of tricyclic anti-depressant overdose**

- Dry skin and mouth
- Urinary retention
- Tachycardia
- Ataxia
- Jerky limb movements
- Divergent squint
- Altered level of consciousness

Opiate excess should be considered in this man who has had access to the simple analgesic co-codamol, which is a combination of paracetamol and the opiate codeine.

Likewise amitriptyline overdose, a common cause of coma, should be considered in the light of his depression and access to the medication. The clinical signs of tricyclic anti-depressant overdose are found in Box 1.3.

Intracranial haemorrhage

Vascular causes of coma are common. This man is known to have hypertension, which puts him at risk of intracranial haemorrhage. The cardinal features of an intracranial haemorrhage are sudden onset of headache, altered consciousness and focal neurological signs. Spontaneous intracranial haemorrhage usually occurs either into the subarachnoid space or into the ventricles and brain substance itself giving rise to either subarachnoid haemorrhage or intra-parenchymal haemorrhage respectively (see Figure 1.1).

Strokes due to cerebral infarction usually present differently to intracranial haemorrhages. The most important difference is that in most strokes consciousness is not impaired. There may be difficulty communicating with the patient, due to expressive or receptive dysphasia, but conscious level itself is not often altered. In brainstem infarctions, which can produce 'locked in syndromes' patients are aware of their surroundings, but unable to respond or communicate, so the patient can appear to be comatose.

Infection

Infection can lead to coma, either systemic infection as in a septicaemic illness, or intracranial infection such as meningitis or encephalitis. Patients with meningitis or encephalitis may present in coma especially if there is raised intracranial pressure.

There will often be a preceding phase characterised by symptoms suggestive of meningeal irritation (stiff neck, headache, photophobia), the signs of raised intracranial pressure (irritability, altered level of consciousness, vomiting, fits) and infection (fever, lethargy). If *Neisseria meningitidis* is the causative organism, the characteristic petechial/purpural rash is seen in approximately 50% of patients

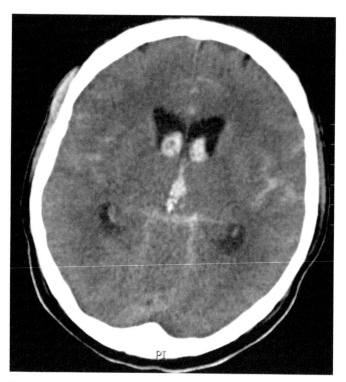

Figure 1.1 Intracranial haemorrhage. CT scan of a patient with an extensive intra-parenchymal haemorrhage. Intra-ventricular blood is seen, as is dilatation of the temporal horns of the lateral ventricles suggesting hydrocephalus.

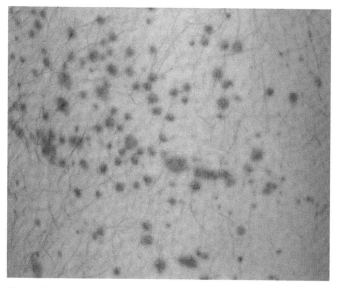

Figure 1.2 Purpuric rash.

(see Figure 1.2); other organisms can cause less well-defined rashes. Other causative organisms can be seen in Table 1.2.

Prompt recognition of the possibility of meningitis is vital, as if left untreated, it has a mortality rate approaching 100%.

This man has a discharging ear infection which could potentially be the source of intracranial infection.

Table 1.2 Causes of meningitis/encephalitis.

Bacterial	*Neisseria meningitidis*, *Streptococcus pneumoniae*, listeria (elderly), *Haemophilus influenzae*, TB
Viral	Herpes simplex, Coxsackie, mumps, echovirus, HIV
Fungal	*Cryptococcus neoformans*
Other	Drugs (trimethoprim/NSAIDs), sarcoidosis, systemic lupus erythematosus

---

Box 1.4 **Atypical clinical signs in coma**

- Intact blink response
- Actively holding eyes closed
- Actively closing eyes when opened
- Presence of Bell's phenomenon (eyes rolled up inside head when observer opens eyes)

Post-ictal state

Following a generalised seizure, patients can be unresponsive as part of a post-ictal state. Typically, though the patient may be in coma immediately following the fit, their conscious level quickly improves within 30–60 minutes, by which time they are usually able to provide you with a history of events. Evidence of urinary incontinence and tongue biting with bleeding in or around the mouth supports the diagnosis but is not diagnostic. The duration of this man's unconscious state would be out of keeping with a post-ictal state.

However, on examination it would be important to look for evidence of ongoing seizure activity (e.g. hypertonicity) as status epilepticus may be a possibility.

Psychogenic coma

Psychogenic coma is uncommon and accounts for less than 2% of all cases of coma and is strictly a diagnosis of exclusion. Accordingly, the patient must be assessed thoroughly to check for other causes of altered consciousness as conditions such as hydrocephalus and vertebral artery dissection have on occasions been initially labelled as psychogenic. There are a number of clinical features that may suggest that the patient is physiologically awake (see Box 1.4) but none could be said to be diagnostic.

Causes of coma not suggested by the history

Trauma

Head injury is one of the commonest causes of coma but this man's history is not suggestive of an intracranial injury.

Structural causes

Structural causes of coma are relatively rare. Intracerebral space-occupying lesions cause coma, either as a result of their mass effect on the brain, or because of the anatomical position of the lesion.

By far the most common cause of cerebral space-occupying lesions are tumours, either primary or secondary. Other causes include cerebral abscess, cysts (e.g. cysticercosis, third ventricular colloid cysts) and granulomas (e.g. sarcoidosis, TB).

Box 1.5 **Metabolic causes of coma**

- Hypoxia
- Hypercapnea (CO_2 narcosis)
- Hypo- or hypercalcaemia
- Hypo- or hypernatraemia
- Uraemia
- Hepatic encephalopathy
- Addison's disease
- Cushing's disease
- Hypo- or hyperthyroidism
- Hypopituitarism

Typically, space-occupying lesions are responsible for slowly progressive symptoms, though it is possible for acute coma to be caused by haemorrhage into a space-occupying lesion.

Carbon monoxide poisoning

Carbon monoxide poisoning is a relatively uncommon cause of coma. Smoke inhalation, fumes from poorly maintained gas appliances and car exhaust fumes are all potential causes. If the poisoning is chronic, prodromal symptoms such as fatigue and headaches may provide clues as to the cause. It is common for members of the same household to be affected, and the lack of symptoms in his wife suggests that this is not the diagnosis.

Metabolic causes

Other metabolic causes not mentioned above are listed in Box 1.5.

Case history revisited

On further questioning, the patient's wife confirmed that he hadn't taken any of the prescribed co-codamol or amitriptyline tablets as the bottles remained full, and that he didn't drink alcohol.

They had a domestic carbon monoxide monitor, which had been checked recently and was in perfect working order.

Examination

Examination of the patient showed him to have a Glasgow Coma Score (GCS) of 7 (E2, M4, V1).

The patient had a clear airway and was breathing with a respiratory rate of 18 per minute.

There was no smell of alcohol or ketones on his breath. Chest auscultation revealed no abnormality. His heart rate was 94 beats/minute and regular, blood pressure was 180/105 mmHg and his temperature was 36.2°C. His bedside blood glucose level was 6.2 mmol/l.

There were no external signs of head injury, and examination of the thorax, abdomen and limbs was unremarkable. There was no visible rash.

His pupils were equally sized and reactive to light. His limbs were generally hypotonic with brisk reflexes on his right upper and lower limbs, with an upgoing right plantar reflex.

management is required to control his blood pressure at this time.

Question: Given the history and examination findings what is your principal working diagnosis?

Principle working diagnosis – Intracerebral haemorrhage

The clinical information given allows us to discount a number of the differential diagnoses.

The patient is not hypoglycaemic and there is no suggestion of opiate or amitriptyline ingestion. He is afebrile and has no evidence of meningococcal disease. The patient's history of hypertension and the acute nature of the onset of coma strongly suggest a vascular cause such as an intracerebral haemorrhage.

Management

This man is in coma and requires an urgent CT scan. As his GCS is 7, his airway is vulnerable and he requires a definitive airway. Intubation and ventilation is required. No specific management is required to control his blood pressure at this time.

Outcome

A CT scan of the patient's brain showed a large intracerebral haemorrhage, with intraventricular blood and hydrocephalus. Urgent neurosurgical advice was sought but unfortunately this man died during an operation to drain his hydrocephalus.

Further reading

Axford J, O'Callaghan C. *Medicine*, Second Edition. Blackwell Science, Oxford, 2004.

Patten JP. *Neurological Differential Diagnosis*. Springer-Verlag, Berlin, 1995.

Ramrakha P, Moore K. *Oxford Handbook of Acute Medicine*, Second Edition. Oxford University Press, Oxford, 2004.

Tintinalli J, Kelen G, Stapczynski S, *et al. Emergency Medicine: A Comprehensive Study Guide*, Sixth Edition. McGraw-Hill, New York, 2003.

Wyatt JP, Illingworth R, Graham C, *et al. Oxford Handbook of Emergency Medicine*, Third Edition. Oxford University Press, Oxford, 2006.

CHAPTER 2

Calf Pain

Francis Morris and Alan Fletcher

CASE HISTORY

A 43-year-old man presents with pain and swelling in his right calf. Three days before he was aware of discomfort and cramping in his right calf associated with some swelling. He took paracetamol but the symptoms continued. On the day of presentation he had slipped on getting out of the shower and developed a pulling sensation in the back of his leg associated with a sudden increase in the amount of pain and consequently he is now walking with a limp. In the past he suffered with ulcerative colitis which was controlled with Salazopyrin and had recently received a course of ciprofloxacin for epididymo-orchitis. He is a smoker but there is no other relevant past medical history. He denies any other symptoms.

Question: What differential diagnosis would you consider from the history?

There are a variety of causes of calf pain which can be divided into those of sudden onset, which frequently have a musculoskeletal origin, and those of an insidious onset, which include important conditions such as deep venous thrombosis (DVT).

Calf muscle injury

One of the commonest problems giving rise to sudden acute pain in the calf is a tear of the medial head of the gastrocnemius muscle (Figure 2.1). This injury is commoner in men and typically occurs in those individuals who are unaccustomed to regular exercise. The injury occurs when the leg is loaded and the person is involved in activities such as running up an incline, jumping or suddenly pushing off as in running for a bus. An audible pop or tearing sensation may be felt in the upper medial aspect of the calf causing the individual to occasionally complain of being struck by a flying object or hit from behind. The patient's calf suddenly becomes painful and full weight bearing is difficult.

Clinical examination reveals localised tenderness to the medial head of the gastrocnemius muscle which may be associated with some swelling. Bruising and discolouration tends to appear days later when it has a tendency to track down the leg to the ankle.

ABC of Emergency Differential Diagnosis. Edited by F. Morris and A. Fletcher.
© 2009 Blackwell Publishing, ISBN: 978-1-4051-7063-5.

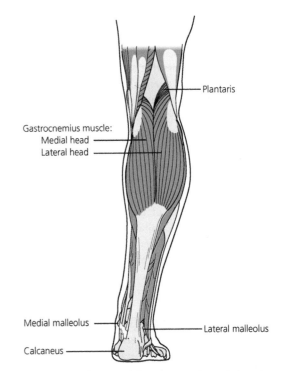

Figure 2.1 Anatomical drawing of the gastrocnemius and plantaris muscle.

Plantaris rupture

The plantaris muscle is a vestigial structure that comprises a small muscular belly and a long tendon. Rupture of this structure will also occur suddenly and painfully but unlike the much commoner gastrocnemius injury the clinical findings are much less specific, hence this is not a diagnosis that will be obvious on clinical examination.

Injury to the plantaris muscle is the diagnosis that one is usually left with when all other common causes of sudden calf pain have been excluded.

Ruptured Baker's cyst

A Baker's cyst is an outpouching of the synovium of the knee joint which occurs in people with an inflammatory or degenerative arthritis (see Figure 2.2). Patients may be aware that they have developed a Baker's cyst because of a fullness in the popliteal fossa behind their knee. When the fluids leaks out of the synovium into the calf muscle it excites an intense inflammatory response giving rise to the sudden onset of pain and swelling.

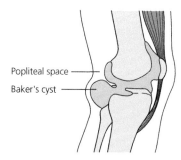

Figure 2.2 Diagram showing a Baker's cyst.

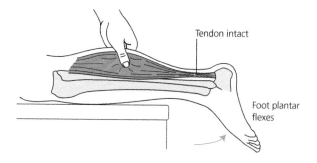

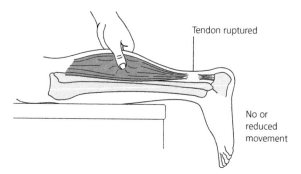

In a typical case the patient will complain of recurrent pain, stiffness and swelling of the knee joint and occasionally they notice how their knee symptoms and signs improve at about the same time as the pain and swelling develops in their calf. The moment of rupture may be felt as a sharp pain behind the knee when the patient is engaged in activities that will increase the pressure within the joint, e.g. squatting, or alternatively the leak may occur more insidiously giving rise to pain and swelling in the calf which may resemble the onset of a DVT.

In some patients there is a joint effusion and/or an obvious full-ness behind the knee joint apparent on palpation. However, the absence of such clinical findings does not exclude the diagnosis.

Figure 2.4 The calf squeeze test.

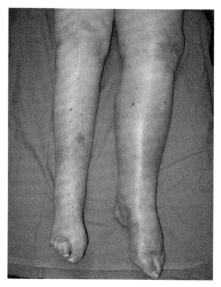

Achilles tendon rupture

Partial or complete rupture of the Achilles tendon occurs sud-denly. As with a calf muscle injury the patient may believe they have been struck from behind by an object or kicked. The usual site of the Achilles tendon rupture, however, is approximately 6 cm above its insertion into the heel bone and therefore the site of pain and discomfort is quite distinct from that of a calf muscle injury (see Figure 2.3).

In a typical case there will be a palpable gap in the Achilles tendon associated with swelling at the site of rupture. Rupture is confirmed clinically by performing the calf squeeze test (see Figure 2.4). When positive, squeezing the calf fails to produce plantar flexion move-ment at the ankle when compared with the normal side.

The patient will still have the ability to actively plantar flex their foot though due to the presence of other intact tendons such as tibialis posterior and flexor hallucis longus, though plantar flexion will be weak. The patient also retains the ability to stand on tiptoes when standing on both feet but they cannot stand on tiptoes using the affected foot alone.

Figure 2.5 A deep venous thrombosis.

Deep venous thrombosis

The signs and symptoms of DVT are related to the degree of obstruction and inflammation of the veins involved. In contrast to calf muscle injuries, the onset is usually insidious with aching, tenderness and swelling developing over a number of days.

Many of the signs are non specific, but oedema of the affected leg is one of the most constant findings (see Figure 2.5).

Redness and warmth may be present over the area of thrombo-sis and as a result the differential diagnosis of a DVT frequently involves cellulitis. DVT is slightly more common in men and individuals over the age of 40.

Factors that promote venous stasis, vessel wall injury or are pro-thrombotic (Virchow's triad) render individuals susceptible to

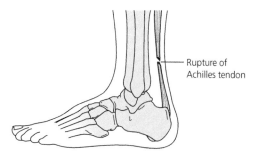

Figure 2.3 Anatomical drawing of the rupture of the Achilles tendon.

the development of DVT. Examples include prolonged immobility, major surgery, thrombophilias.

Other causes of calf pain not suggested by the history

Referred pain from the back

Patients with radicular symptoms associated with degenerative back problems may present with what appears to be isolated calf pain. The lack of localised signs apart from tenderness or hypersensitivity, a history of back problems and the findings that the symptoms are exacerbated by straight leg raising would all point to a diagnosis of referred pain from the back.

Thrombophlebitis

Discrete tenderness and thread like lumpiness overlying the superficial vein may give rise to the complaint of calf pain. Remember, however, that superficial thrombophlebitis in the absence of varicose veins is a risk factor for DVT.

Popliteal aneurysm

A contained haemorrhage from a popliteal aneurysm into the calf muscle may give rise to the sudden onset of pain and discomfort which may present in a similar fashion to a calf muscle tear or a ruptured Baker's cyst. This is a rare complication of aneurysmal disease. The diagnosis should be considered if any patient presents with the sudden onset of calf pain in association with a popliteal aneurysm.

Arterial insufficiency

It is well recognised that chronic arterial insufficiency gives rise to calf pain on exertion, which is relieved by rest. Acute arterial insufficiency will result in rest pain, though these symptoms are rarely isolated to the calf. Hence, acute vascular insufficiency does not usually form part of the differential diagnosis of calf pain.

Cellulitis

Cellulitis gives rise to red, tender, painful, swollen lower legs but as with arterial insufficiency the condition is rarely isolated to the calf. Given the non-specific way in which DVT can present, cellulitis is frequently considered in the differential diagnosis of this condition but not in the differential diagnosis of isolated calf pain.

Case history revisited

Revisiting the presenting symptoms, the diagnosis is not immediately obvious. This man's history is not entirely compatible with a calf muscle injury as three days prior to the sudden pain he complained of swelling and tenderness in his calf. The insidious onset of pain and swelling in his calf suggests that leaking from a Baker's cyst or DVT should be considered.

He has a minor risk factor in ulcerative colitis but no major risk factors for a DVT though the fact that he is taking ciprofloxacin (which is associated with spontaneous rupture of the Achilles tendon) is worth noting.

Examination

Clinical examination reveals no obvious limitation of movement of his right knee joint, pain, tenderness or effusion. His temperature is normal.

There is no localised tenderness over the medial head of his gastrocnemius muscle nor any bruising to his calf. The calf squeeze test reveals that his Achilles tendon function is intact and there is no neurovascular deficit.

Question: Given the history and examination findings what is your principal working diagnosis?

Principal working diagnosis – DVT

Management

Given the non-specific way in which a DVT may present and the fact that a number of conditions may give rise to similar symptoms, the investigation of a patient with a possible DVT is informed by assessing their pre-test probability.

The Wells clinical prediction guide (see Table 2.1) or a modification of the same is frequently used. This guide uses a number of risk factors and clinical findings to allow the patient to be graded as high or low probability for DVT. It is important when scoring a patient using such a guide that appropriate attention is given to any alternative diagnosis that is as, or more, likely than a DVT. It is important that this category is assessed correctly to prevent the patient being given a falsely high pre-test probability resulting in them undergoing unnecessary investigations.

It is now also common practice to measure the D-dimer levels in any individuals at low risk of DVT. D-dimer fragments are present in fresh clots and in fibrin degradation products and therefore elevated in many conditions where blood clots develop, including DVT. The combination of the pre-test probability and the D-dimer result help inform the investigation strategy.

Table 2.1 Pre-test probability assessment for DVT.

Clinical features	Score
Malignancy (treatment ongoing in last 6 months or palliative)	1
Paralysis, paresis, recent plaster immobilisation lower limb	1
Recently bedridden >3 days or major surgery within 12 weeks	1
Entire leg swollen	1
Localised tenderness along distribution of deep venous system	1
Calf diameter more than 3 cm greater than asymptomatic leg	1
Pitting oedema (confined to symptomatic leg)	1
Colateral superficial veins (non-varicose)	1
Previous documented DVT	1
Alternative diagnosis at least as likely as that of DVT	−2
Pre-Test probability of DVT	
Unlikely: 1 or less	
Likely: 2 or more	

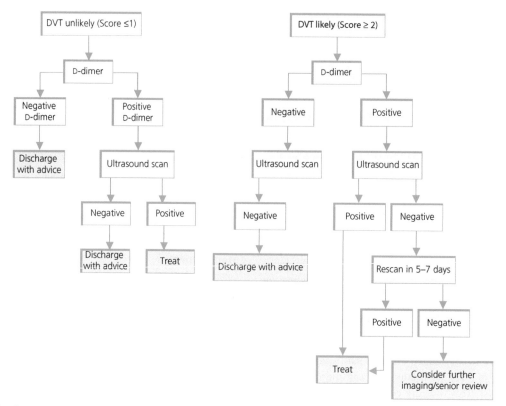

Figure 2.6 Algorithm for investigation of suspected deep vein thrombosis: Application of clinical model to pre-test probability.

The commonest form of imaging used to identify a DVT is duplex ultrasound which has a sensitivity for proximal vein DVT of 97% and a negative predictive value of 95%. Impedance plethysmography is an alternative non-invasive technique used in some centres. Venography, which is invasive, is not often performed today, and now is only considered in high risk patients when ultrasound examinations have been inconclusive. An alternative to venography is MRI angiography which is expensive, though becoming increasingly available. An investigation strategy is seen in Figure 2.6.

Ultrasound is very helpful in diagnosing other causes of calf pain, especially Baker's cyst and Achilles tendon rupture.

Blood tests are rarely helpful in assisting diagnosis, though a raised white cell count points towards cellulitis.

Outcome

This man was assessed as having a pre-test probability of +2 as his calf was swollen and there was tenderness over the deep venous system. There was no other obvious diagnosis and therefore the minus two category did not apply in this case. In addition his D-dimer test was elevated.

A duplex ultrasound scan revealed a non-occlusive blood clot in the superficial femoral vein of his thigh.

Further reading

Donnelly R, London NJM. *ABC of Arterial and Venous Disease.* Blackwell Science, Oxford, 2000.

Tintinalli J, Kelen G, Stapczynski S, *et al. Emergency Medicine: A Comprehensive Study Guide,* Sixth Edition. McGraw-Hill, New York, 2003.

Wardrope J, English B. *Musculo-Skeletal Problems in Emergency Medicine.* Oxford University Press, Oxford, 1998.

Wyatt JP, Illingworth R, Graham C, *et al. Oxford Handbook of Emergency Medicine,* Third Edition. Oxford University Press, Oxford, 2006.

CHAPTER 3

Chest Pain – Cardiac

Nicki Doddridge

CASE HISTORY

A 47-year-old man presents with chest pain. He has noticed the pain over the past few weeks with strenuous activity. He describes an ache in the centre of his chest associated with mild dyspnoea. The patient first noticed the pain whilst climbing a ladder at work. Since then it has occurred on several occasions whilst walking up the hill to his local newsagents. This morning he was playing football with his son when it began. It was a little more severe than usual and this time he had an ache in his left shoulder. Usually the pain resolves quickly when he stops what he is doing. This morning it lasted about 30 minutes. He works as a labourer on a building site and this week has been moving heavy flagstones. He stopped smoking 2 years ago after his father died of a heart attack. He drinks 40 units of alcohol per week and has a 15 pack-year smoking history. His GP recently started him on lansoprazole 15 mg after he complained of a burning sensation in his chest. The pain he was prescribed this for was a little different. It was more of a burning sensation in bed at night. This has subsided somewhat since he started treatment. He still gets occasional symptoms, however, after overindulging in rich foods.

Question: What differential diagnosis would you consider from the history?

The differential diagnosis of chest pain is very wide, with many possible causes (see Box 3.1). With careful history taking it is usually possible to narrow the diagnosis, and in this case three differential diagnoses are prominent.

Angina pectoris

Chest pain deservedly receives so much attention and importance because ischaemic heart disease (IHD) often manifests with this symptom. Unfortunately, classical symptoms of central, crushing chest pain that radiates to the neck, jaw and left arm are not always obvious. Patients often describe a 'sharp' pain, and pain may be felt in the epigastrium or left arm only. Frustratingly, some patients with clear evidence of IHD have no symptoms whatsoever. Typically, the diagnosis of angina is made when pain develops on exertion, and

Box 3.1 **Causes of chest pain**

Cardiac
- Angina
- Acute coronary syndrome
- Myocarditis/pericarditis
- Arrhythmia
- Mitral valve prolapse

Gastrointestinal
- Gastro-oesophageal reflux
- Peptic ulcer disease
- Pancreatitis
- Hepatobiliary

Vascular
- Thoracic aortic dissection

Respiratory
- Pneumothorax
- Pneumonia
- Pulmonary embolism
- Neoplasia
- Hyperventilation

Musculoskeletal
- Muscular strain
- Direct chest wall injury
- Rib fracture
- Costochondritis/Tietze's disease

Other
- Herpes zoster infection

Box 3.2 **Risk factors for IHD**

- Smoking
- Advancing age
- Hypercholesterolaemia
- Hypertension
- Diabetes mellitus
- Male sex
- Abdominal obesity (high waist–hip ratio)
- Family history

settles with rest. Pain that comes on at rest, is rapidly worsening, or is linked with ECG changes of myocardial damage usually represents an acute coronary syndrome. This used to be divided into unstable angina and myocardial infarction but it is usual now to consider all of these conditions as different points in a spectrum of coronary artery disease.

To help with diagnosis, risk factors for IHD should be sought (see Box 3.2). The likelihood of IHD increases when three or more factors are present. History that indicates another cause should be considered carefully, but the bottom line is that IHD should be a principal diagnosis to initially exclude in most cases of undifferentiated chest pain.

ABC of Emergency Differential Diagnosis. Edited by F. Morris and A. Fletcher.
© 2009 Blackwell Publishing, ISBN: 978-1-4051-7063-5.

Physical examination is usually normal, but becomes important if signs indicate aortic stenosis or hypertrophic cardiomyopathy (ejection systolic murmur, pulse character abnormalities).

Musculoskeletal chest pain

Musculoskeletal chest pain is common, but because the risks associated with it are small, the diagnosis is usually made when other more serious causes have been excluded. A history of injury or unaccustomed exertion is important and costochondritis may be associated with systemic viral illness symptoms. Examination may show reproducible chest wall tenderness or pain on movement. Be aware that pressing on the chest wall usually feels sore in normal people, and one must be very clear about the relationship of thoracic rotation to the presenting pain symptom.

Gastro-oesophageal reflux

Another common cause of chest pain, this is classically described as a burning sensation behind the sternum, aggravated by supine posture. It is linked to high alcohol intake, obesity, and anti-inflammatory drugs. Nicotine also increases the incidence of reflux by causing relaxation of the lower oesophageal sphincter. Unfortunately, there are many similarities between the pain of gastro-oesophageal reflux and IHD; acid reflux has even been shown to cause coronary artery spasm.

Other causes of chest pain not suggested by the history

Aortic dissection

A rare but very significant diagnosis, this is suggested by a severe tearing pain, often between the shoulder blades. Patients may have a difference between the upper limb pulses or blood pressure in the arms. A chest X-ray may show an abnormal aortic arch or a wide mediastinum (Figure 3.1).

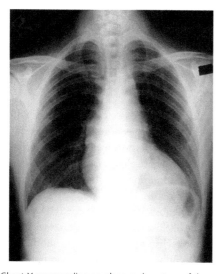

Figure 3.1 Chest X-ray revealing an abnormal contour of the mediastinum and an enlarged heart in a patient with aortic dissection.

Lung causes

Lung cancer, pulmonary embolus, pneumonia, and exacerbations of chronic obstructive pulmonary disease can all cause chest pain. History taking should identify important features reflecting these diagnoses, and a chest X-ray will usually be abnormal.

Case history revisited

This man describes an aching pain in his chest with exertion, associated with dyspnoea. He has been a smoker and there is a family history of IHD. These are important features pointing towards angina as the most likely diagnosis.

Musculoskeletal chest pain is possible because he has a manual job that involves heavy lifting and he may have sustained a muscular injury. We know that he has recently been lifting heavy flagstones and need to know if his pain was present before then. Nevertheless, musculoskeletal pain is a diagnosis of exclusion in this case.

Gastro-oesophageal reflux is possible, but the character of the pain and relationship to exertion make this less likely.

Examination

On examination he is now pain free, his pulse is 90 beats/minute, blood pressure 140/85 mmHg, respiratory rate 14/minute, and oxygen saturations 97% on air. His heart sounds are normal with no murmurs. Chest examination is normal. Abdominal examination reveals centripetal obesity, without organomegaly or tenderness. The pain cannot be reproduced by either palpation of the chest wall or movement of the torso.

Question: Given the history and examination findings what is your principal working diagnosis?

Principal working diagnosis – stable angina pectoris

The absence of alternative diagnostic clues on examination, along with normal observations, points to IHD as the most likely diagnosis. Obesity is an independent risk factor in its own right for IHD, and in isolation does not make gastro-oesophageal reflux likely.

Management

The cornerstone of investigation is the ECG. A 12 lead ECG should be performed promptly in all patients presenting to the Accident and Emergency Department with chest pain. The ECG is performed to assess the presence of detectable myocardial ischaemia or infarction (see Figure 3.2). It is also used to exclude alternative diagnoses such as an arrhythmia, pericarditis or pulmonary embolism. Most patients with a pulmonary embolism will have a normal ECG or sinus tachycardia. The classical changes are of right heart strain, namely S1, Q3, T3 pattern and right bundle branch block. Atrial fibrillation may also be seen. The initial ECG may be normal in up to 20% of patients who go on to receive a diagnosis of IHD.

Blood tests are important for assessing risk and furthering diagnosis for most patients with acute chest pain. Anaemia may unmask

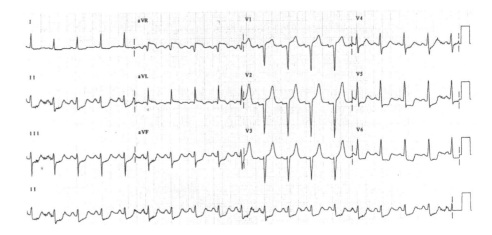

Figure 3.2 ECGs showing ischaemia.

IHD. Haemoglobin concentration and platelets should be assessed when commencing antithrombotic therapies. A raised white cell count may indicate recent infection but may also be raised in response to acute myocardial infarction. Uraemia may be a cause of pericarditis, and abnormal liver function tests may lead to an alternative diagnosis.

Cardiac markers are used to assess myocardial damage. They are released from skeletal as well as cardiac smooth muscle. Therefore, they may also be raised due to trauma and skeletal muscle injury. Elevated levels of troponin indicate myocardial necrosis. Although originally thought to be very specific for myocardial damage due to acute coronary syndrome, troponin may also be released from cardiac myofibrils under other circumstances such as pulmonary oedema, pulmonary embolism, sepsis, myocarditis, arrhythmia and strenuous exertion. Troponin is usually measured 12 hours after the onset of pain but some centres are measuring Troponin at 6 hours along with change in creatinine isoenzyme and same day exercise stress testing.

Chest X-ray should be performed to exclude other pathology. If cardiac markers and ECG are normal, then the patient should proceed to exercise testing as there are no contraindications (see Box 3.3). This is performed with the patient walking on a treadmill with simultaneous heart rate, blood pressure and 12 lead ECG monitoring. The speed and gradient of the treadmill increase every 3 minutes on a standard Bruce protocol. The aim is to increase cardiac work and oxygen demand thus unmasking IHD (see Figure 3.3).

Outcome

A diagnosis of stable angina pectoris with an early positive exercise test was made after the patient exercised for 3 minutes and 50 seconds achieving 74% of his maximum predicted heart rate for age. The test was terminated due to onset of chest pain followed shortly afterwards by ST depression in leads V4–V6, reaching 2 mm of downsloping ST depression at maximum.

The diagnosis was explained and he was prescribed aspirin 75 mg daily, atenolol 50 mg daily and simvastatin 40 mg daily. He was provided with a glyceryl trinitrate (GTN) spray and given instructions on its use. He was also given instructions to dial 999 if he develops chest pain that is unrelieved by his GTN spray. He was counselled

---

Box 3.3 **Contraindications to exercise testing**

Absolute
- Recent acute myocardial infarction (48 hours)
- Ongoing unstable angina
- Arrhythmia causing compromise
- Severe aortic stenosis
- Acute pulmonary embolus
- Acute myocarditis or pericarditis
- Aortic dissection

Relative
- Left main stem stenosis
- Moderate aortic stenosis
- Electrolyte abnormalities
- Severe hypertension (SBP >200, DBP >110 mmHg)
- Hypertrophic cardiomyopathy
- High AV block
- Physical inability to exercise

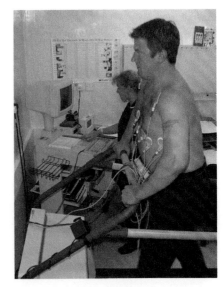

Figure 3.3 Exercise tolerance test in progress.

on risk factor modification and given follow up in the Rapid Access Chest Pain Clinic for consideration for angiography/percutaneous coronary intervention.

Further reading

Axford J, O'Callaghan C. *Medicine*, Second Edition. Blackwell, Oxford, 2004.

Swanton RH, Banerjee S. *Cardiology*, Fifth Edition. Blackwell, Oxford, 2008

Ramrakha P, Moore K. *Oxford Handbook of Acute Medicine*, Second Edition. Oxford University Press, Oxford, 2004.

Simon C, Everitt, H & Kendrick, T. *Oxford Handbook of General Practice*, Second Edition. Oxford University Press, Oxford, 2002.

Wyatt JP, Illingworth R, Graham C, *et al. Oxford Handbook of Emergency Medicine*, Third Edition. Oxford University Press, Oxford, 2006.

CHAPTER 4

High Fever

Rachel Foster

CASE HISTORY

A 29-year-old businessman presents 3 days after returning from a 3 week trip to India with a 56 hour history of headache, abdominal pain, profound malaise and a high fever. He received a course of vaccinations before his trip including Japanese B encephalitis, typhoid, tetanus, diphtheria and polio boosters, rabies and hepatitis A+B. He had taken chloroquine and proguanil as malarial prophylaxis, but had a missed a couple of doses, and had been aware of a few insect bites during his visit. He recalls having drunk mainly bottled water and drinks from bars, some of which contained ice. He denies having sex whilst abroad. He has no significant past medical history and takes no medicines regularly. There is no relevant family history, and he is a single non-smoker who drinks approximately 21 units of alcohol per week.

Question: What differential diagnosis would you consider from the history?

The differential diagnosis of fever, particularly in the returning traveller, is very wide. Finding the diagnosis can be difficult given the non-specific nature of many of the accompanying symptoms, and confirmation often depends upon the results of microbiological or serological tests, which take time. Acquiring a detailed history is invaluable as it can provide important clues. Some of these infections can be rapidly fatal while others have a more indolent course. Viral infections such as influenza A or B or enterovirus are commonly acquired on the aircraft home and must be considered. We will focus on the four most likely serious diagnoses for this case, but be aware that there are many possible diagnoses not suggested by the specific associated symptoms in this case which present with fever (see Table 4.1).

Malaria

Malaria is one of the most common travel-related infections in tropical and sub-tropical areas. It causes around 400–900 million cases of fever and approximately 1–3 million deaths per year worldwide. It is for this reason that malaria should feature in the list of differential diagnoses in nearly all cases of fever in patients returning from endemic areas. The clinical features of malaria include fever (which may or may not be cyclical), malaise and myalgia, headache, anorexia, and anaemia. If severe (usually *Plasmodium falciparum* malaria) then there may also be hypoxia, adult respiratory distress syndrome (ARDS), renal failure, hepatitis, hypoglycaemia, confusion or even coma. The incubation period is usually 7–14 days but may be as long as 1 year, particularly in the context of chemoprophylaxis. It is important not to assume that travellers to their native country are immune – immunity wanes rapidly with time spent away from a malarious area. Also, don't be put off the diagnosis in those who have taken chemoprophylaxis – it remains a possibility.

Examination may reveal pallor, jaundice, hepatosplenomegaly, hypotension, cyanosis and haematuria, or none of the above. The spectrum of disease severity is very wide.

Meningitis

Meningitis is characterised by headache accompanied by photophobia and neck stiffness, high fever, rigors, malaise and profound lethargy, and sometimes a non-blanching rash (variable: tiny petechiae to large necrosing patches – see Figure 4.4). Patients (particularly with meningococcal sepsis) may rapidly develop septic shock. A significant proportion of those with meningococcal sepsis will *not* have meningitis (i.e. no headache/neck stiffness) but their mortality is just as high. In the elderly, listeria meningitis may present as reduced consciousness or confusion without marked meningism. Pneumococcal meningitis may be preceded by sore throat or earache, may have a slower presentation, and should be considered early.

Pneumonia

Fever, rigors, malaise, anorexia, breathlessness, cough and pleuritic chest pain are all common features of pneumonia. Misleading symptoms can include abdominal pain, diarrhoea, jaundice and headache. Recent travel, severe disease, non-respiratory symptoms and deranged liver function strongly indicate *Legionella* as a differential diagnosis. A rapid onset of symptoms plus haemoptysis (often in the absence of initial X-ray changes, sometimes following a soft tissue infection), suggests Panton-Valentine leukocidin (PVL) producing *Staphylococcus aureus* and the microbiology department should be contacted urgently. A long history including cough, haemoptysis, night sweats and weight loss should prompt

ABC of Emergency Differential Diagnosis. Edited by F. Morris and A. Fletcher.
© 2009 Blackwell Publishing, ISBN: 978-1-4051-7063-5.

Table 4.1 Other infections which should be considered in the patient presenting with fever.

Diagnoses	Clinical features	Defining investigations
Septicaemia	Rigors, high fever and chills, malaise, profound muscle weakness, dizziness and confusion	Blood cultures
Cellulitis	Red, hot, tender swollen skin. May have systemic symptoms of sepsis	Blood cultures and skin swabs occasionally define the organism
Epstein–Barr virus (EBV)/streptococcal throat infection	Pustular tonsils may not be obvious until day 2 or 3 of a febrile illness with significant malaise, anorexia and moderate headache (see Figure 4.1)	Throat swab. Monospot test and EBV serology
Lyme disease	Classic erythema chronicum migrans rash in early infection (see Figure 4.2). Cranial nerve palsy, arthritis and heart block in late infection	*Borrelia burgdorferi* serology (on blood or cerebrospinal fluid)
Amoebic liver abscess	Recent dysentery (only 50%), right upper quadrant pain and tenderness and high fever (see Figure 4.3)	Abdominal ultrasound scan/CT scan, amoebic serology. Consider aspiration of collection – pyogenic abscess must urgently be excluded
HIV seroconversion	Sore throat, rash, fever, myalgia. Recent risk behaviour (may not be offered initially)	Low CD4 count, HIV antibody tests may be negative initially. Antigen tests and PCR can be helpful if suspicion is high
Trypanosomiasis	Hepatosplenomegaly, fever, lymphadenopathy Appropriate travel history. Black fly bites	Blood film, serology
Leishmaniasis	Cutaneous ulcer, or hepatosplenomegaly and fever. Travel to Mediterranean, Asia or Africa. Sand fly bites	Blood culture, microscopy of ulcer, bone marrow aspirate and microscopy
Schistosomiasis	Haematuria and dysuria or blood-streaked stool, lethargy. Rash with fever. History of swimming in freshwater lakes in the tropics	Urine and stool microscopy for ova, cysts and parasites. Serology
Various helminth infections	Fever, rash, cough, altered bowel habit. Some related to eating raw fish or other food from endemic areas	Eosinophilia, stool and sputum microscopy for ova, cysts and parasites
SARS and avian influenza	Fever, cough, breathlessness, myalgia, malaise, possible diarrhoea with appropriate travel history in context or current outbreak*	Nasopharyngeal aspirate, serology, electronmicroscopy of respiratory secretions
Viral haemorrhagic fever	Fever, myalgia, malaise, bleeding from gums/nose etc. History of travel to outbreak area, or contact with known case[†]	Viral culture, serology and PCR. Must exclude malaria
Other tick and mosquito-borne spirochetes and viruses, e.g. tick typhus, West Nile virus, Chikungunya, Ross River Fever	Fever, myalgia, arthritis, headache. Travel to endemic areas (outbreaks of West Nile in the USA, and Chikungunya in South Europe)	Serology

*NB, At the time of writing there have not been any human–human transmitted cases of SARS since July 2003. Avian influenza is not transmissible between humans and has only been found in those with close contact with poultry, largely in South-East Asia. Although there have been incidences of avian influenza in British poultry, there have not been any human cases as yet.

[†]Suspected cases of viral haemorrhagic fever must be isolated and managed by staff wearing personal protection equipment until a risk assessment has been made by a specialist.

investigation for acid fast bacilli and TB culture. The patient should be isolated if chest X-ray changes are typical (see Figure 4.5).

Typhoid/paratyphoid

'Enteric fever' is caused by *Salmonella enterica* serovars Typhi, and Paratyphi types A, B and C with an incubation period of 7–14 days. Typhoid and paratyphoid are endemic in many parts of the tropics where ice and frozen dairy products, in addition to other foodstuffs, are often contaminated with the bacteria. Paratyphoid usually causes a clinically milder illness than typhoid.

Patients present with persistently high fever, headache, malaise, lethargy, apathy, anorexia, nausea and often abdominal pain. Early in the illness patients may describe constipation, with diarrhoea occurring later. Neuropsychiatric complications occur late. Sometimes a relative bradycardia is noted, but is not universal. Generalised abdominal pain may be accompanied by liver and spleen enlargement. Rose spots (pink macular/maculopapular blanching lesions) may be found on the trunk (see Figure 4.6) in patients with typhoid. Crackles may be heard bi-basally in the chest. Increasing girth size and pain may indicate ileal perforation.

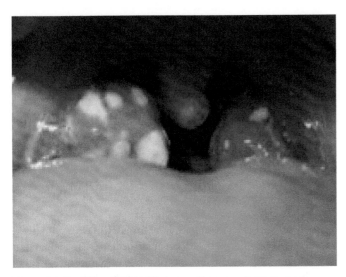

Figure 4.1 Tonsillitis – typical of that caused by group A streptococcus. Image courtesy of www.answers.com/topic/tonsillitis?cat=health

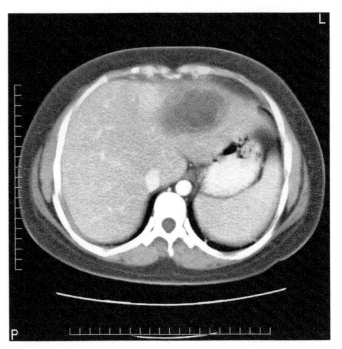

Figure 4.3 Amoebic liver abscess. Image courtesy of www.medicine.mcgill.ca/tropmed/txt/lecture1%20intest%20protozoa.htm/amoebabscess.jpg

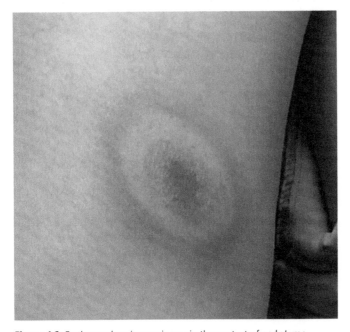

Figure 4.2 Erythema chronicum migrans in the context of early Lyme disease. Image courtesy of mdchoice.com.bmp

Other causes of high fever not suggested by the history

There are many illnesses other than infections of which fever is a prominent symptom. Examples are given in Box 4.1. In this case the history of travel is especially relevant and infections must be considered. In other cases of fever, infections feature as or less importantly in the differential diagnosis.

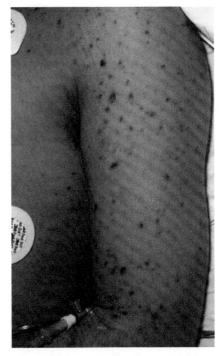

Figure 4.4 Meningococcal rash. Image kindly provided by Doctors mess, www.doctors.net.uk

Case history revisited

On revisiting the patient's history the diagnosis is still not clear. The history of headache is worrying but not specific for meningitis. Abdominal pain is more indicative of enteric fever, but we need to know more about whether the patient has suffered from

diarrhoea or constipation. Malaria is distinctly possible, as it could explain all the symptoms and requires urgent diagnostic consideration. Vaccination offers protection against *Salmonella* Typhi, but consequently only confers immunity against one form of enteric fever, and only if a person maintains appropriate antibody titres.

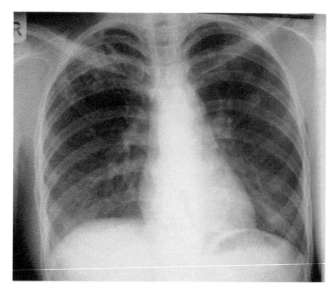

Figure 4.5 Pulmonary tuberculosis. Image kindly provided by Dr Andrew McDonald Johnston, www.doctors.net.uk

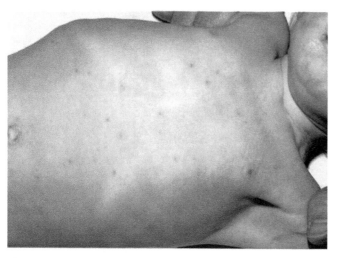

Figure 4.6 Rose spots in the context of typhoid. Image courtesy of the Health Protection Agency via Doctors mess, www.doctors.net.uk

Box 4.1 **Non-infective causes of fever**

- Malignancy
- Autoimmune diseases
- Drug reactions – allergic reactions to, or metabolic consequences of the drug
- Seizures
- Environmental fever (due to very high external temperatures, or excessive exercise)
- Hyperthyroidism
- Thrombosis
- Infarction – of myocardium, kidney, or lung (auto-immune element)
- Blood transfusion reaction
- Atmospheric pollution (e.g. nitrogen dioxide)
- Factitious fever (Munchausen's syndrome/Munchausen's by proxy)

The possibility of typhoid or paratyphoid in particular is possible given a relatively low efficacy of the vaccine (55–70%) and the history of ice consumption.

Examination

Observations are as follows: blood pressure 90/60 mmHg, pulse 60 beats/min, temperature 38.9°C, respiratory rate 20 breaths/min, oxygen saturations 98% on air. On general examination he appears unwell and lethargic with a greyish pallor. He is not jaundiced; there is no evidence of anaemia, lymphadenopathy, clubbing or cyanosis. There are a couple of blanching, pink maculae on his flank, but otherwise no evidence of rash on his skin.

There are fine crackles in both lung bases. His JVP is not visible. Heart sounds are normal, with no ankle oedema. His abdomen is soft but generally tender. The tip of the liver can just be felt, but no other organomegaly or masses are palpable. Bowel sounds are present. He is neurologically fully intact with a Glasgow Coma Score of 15/15. Fundoscopy is normal and he has no neck stiffness.

Question: Given the history and examination findings what is your principal working diagnosis?

Principal working diagnosis – enteric fever

Malaria is still possible. Hypotension and his lethargic, unwell appearance point to this, but the absence of jaundice, pronounced pallor or hepatosplenomegaly casts doubt. Meningitis is unlikely as the headache is not accompanied by meningism. Septicaemia of some type is still possible. Amoebic liver abscess might be a possibility, although one would expect more pronounced right upper quadrant pain and tenderness. The lack of respiratory symptoms or signs makes pneumonia unlikely. Enteric fever is much more likely given the presence of pink macules (possible rose spots), accompanied by diffuse abdominal tenderness, mild anaemia and mild hepatitis, and a heart rate of 60 in a febrile patient.

Management

This patient requires urgent fluid resuscitation and oxygen. Investigation includes full blood count, renal and liver function tests, ESR, CRP and chest X-ray. Three thick blood films specifically for malaria parasites and haemolysis should be sent urgently. Blood, urine, and stool should be cultured. If these do not yield a result, bone marrow aspirate culture should be considered. Do not request a Widal test for typhoid; it has been abandoned by most laboratories in the UK due to difficulty in the interpretation of results. Your laboratory may have the newer rapid antigen tests available. Urinary antigen testing should be performed if *Legionella* is suspected.

If meningitis is suspected in the absence of a classic meningococcal rash, a lumbar puncture should be performed to confirm the diagnosis and identify the organism unless contraindicated. If the history and examination point to pneumococcal meningitis a dose of steroids with the first dose of antibiotics can improve outcome.

As enteric fever is likely, treatment with i.v. ceftriaxone or cefotaxime should be initiated whilst awaiting the microbiological results and sensitivity testing. The patient may require inotropic support. Management in an infectious diseases unit is appropriate.

Outcome

This patient's investigations showed negative malaria films, mild anaemia, lymphopaenia, mild abnormalities of liver function and a normal chest X-ray. His ESR was 87 and CRP 264. *Salmonella* Typhi subsequently grew on stool culture. He was managed in an infectious diseases unit with fluids and intravenous ceftriaxone, and was monitored for development of ileal perforation by measuring girth size. He made a full recovery.

Further reading

Connor BA, Schwartz E. Typhoid and paratyphoid fever in travellers. *Lancet Infectious Diseases* 2005; **5**:623–628.

Cook GC (Ed.). *Manson's Tropical Diseases*, 21st Edition. Saunders, London, 2003.

Felton JM, Bryceson AD. Fever in the returning traveller. *British Journal of Hospital Medicine* 1996; **55**:705–711.

Health Protection Agency website: www.hpa.org.uk

Heyderman RS on behalf of the British Infection Society. Early management of suspected bacterial meningitis and meningococcal septicaemia in immunocompetent adults. *Journal of Infection* 2005; **50**:373–374. Also www.meningitis.org

Lalloo DG, Shingadia D, Pasvol G *et al.* UK malaria treatment guidelines. *Journal of Infection* 2007; **54**:111–121.

Ledingham JG, Warrell DA. *Concise Oxford Textbook of Medicine*. Oxford University Press, Oxford, 2000.

Spira AM. Assessment of travellers who return home ill. *Lancet* 2003; **361**:1459–1469. www.britishinfectionsociety.org

www.dh.gov.uk/en/Publichealth/Healthprotection/Immunisation/Greenbook/DH_4097254. Immunisation against Infectious Disease – 'the Green Book'. www.wrongdiagnosis.com/f/fever/causes.htm

CHAPTER 5

Vaginal Bleeding

Sian Ireland and Karen Selby

CASE HISTORY

A 36-year-old, obese, diabetic woman presents with a 5-day history of heavy vaginal bleeding. She is passing clots and using more than 10 pads per day. The bleeding is accompanied by right-sided lower abdominal pain that is constant and becoming more severe. She has not vomited but has lost her appetite. In her early twenties she was treated for a sexually transmitted infection. She has a long history of irregular periods attributed to polycystic ovary syndrome (PCOS), and has previously tried clomiphene in order to try to become pregnant. Her last menstrual period was 8 weeks ago but given her menstrual irregularity she is not overly concerned by this. She is sexually active and is not using any contraception. She has no other medical problems and there is no family history of a tendency to bleed.

Box 5.1 **Causes of vaginal bleeding**

Non-pregnant
- Dysfunctional uterine bleeding
- Cervical erosion
- Cervical polyps
- Infection
- Malignancy

Early pregnancy
- Spontaneous miscarriage
- Ectopic pregnancy

Late pregnancy
- Placental abruption
- Placenta praevia

Question: What differential diagnosis would you consider from the history?

The differential diagnosis of heavy vaginal bleeding is listed in Box 5.1.

This woman could be pregnant as she has not had a period for 8 weeks. Bleeding in early pregnancy is most often due to a miscarriage, but ectopic pregnancy is the other important diagnosis to consider.

Miscarriage

Spontaneous miscarriage is the loss of a pregnancy before 24 weeks gestation. It is thought that around 10–20% of pregnancies result in spontaneous miscarriage. The majority are due to embryonic abnormalities with a small percentage attributable to maternal health factors such as diabetes, renal disease, autoimmune disorders, trauma and infections, or structural abnormalities of the reproductive tract (see Figure 5.1).

1 Threatened miscarriage. This is vaginal bleeding during early pregnancy without the passage of tissue. The cervical os remains closed and a viable pregnancy is seen in the uterus. About half will progress to an actual miscarriage.

The bleeding and accompanying pain is not usually severe, and on vaginal examination the os is closed and there is no cervical excitation.

2 Inevitable miscarriage. There is dilatation of the cervical canal and bleeding is usually more severe.

3 Incomplete miscarriage. Vaginal bleeding is more intense and accompanied by abdominal pain. On vaginal examination the os is open and tissue is being passed. The presence of tissue in the os itself can cause cervical shock – low blood pressure accompanied by bradycardia due to vagal stimulation. If the tissue is removed with sponge forceps the shock will usually resolve.

4 Complete miscarriage. This is said to have occurred when the fetus and the entire placenta have been passed. There is a history of vaginal bleeding and pain which has usually subsided. Ultrasound scan reveals an empty uterus.

5 Delayed or missed miscarriage. This can only be diagnosed by ultrasound scan when a gestational sac with a mean diameter of more than 20 mm is seen but there is no fetal pole, or a fetal pole greater than 6 mm is present but no fetal heart pulsation is detected. These may present with slight vaginal bleeding.

Ectopic pregnancy

This occurs when a fertilised ovum implants at a site other than in the uterus. Most often it occurs in the fallopian tubes but also occur within the abdomen, cervix or ovary (see Box 5.2 and Figure 5.2).

ABC of Emergency Differential Diagnosis. Edited by F. Morris and A. Fletcher. © 2009 Blackwell Publishing, ISBN: 978-1-4051-7063-5.

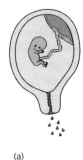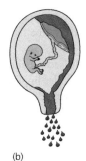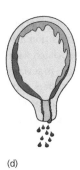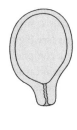

Figure 5.1 Miscarriage. (a) Threatened. (b) Inevitable. (c) Complete. (d) Incomplete.

(a) (b) (c) (d)

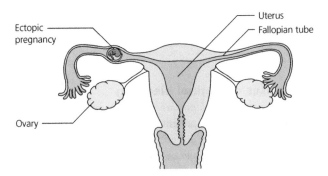

Uterus
Fallopian tube
Ectopic pregnancy
Ovary

Figure 5.2 Ectopic pregnancy.

The incidence is thought to be around 1–2% of reported pregnancies, and is increasing. Ectopic pregnancies account for 8% of direct maternal deaths in the Confidential Enquiry into Maternal and Child Health. The condition most commonly occurs in the 25–34 years age group.

There is usually a history of a late period and abdominal or pelvic pain. Vaginal bleeding is usually minimal but can be severe in the rare cases of cervical ectopic pregnancy. The presence of shoulder pain suggests diaphragmatic irritation by free peritoneal fluid from a ruptured ectopic pregnancy. There may be shock.

Clinical examination unfortunately is unreliable. If pregnancy testing is positive an ultrasound scan may confirm the presence of an intra- or extrauterine pregnancy. However, this may not be possible.

In a shocked patient, rapid resuscitation and urgent referral to a gynaecologist is necessary. Laparotomy is usually performed but laparoscopy may be possible with a skilled operator. The priority is to identify and control the point of haemorrhage. Typically the source of bleeding is at the site where the ectopic pregnancy has ruptured through a fallopian tube. In these cases partial salpingectomy may be appropriate.

In a haemodynamically stable patient the surgical route of choice is laparoscopy. Salpingectomy is usually performed but it may be possible to attempt to conserve the tube by performing a salpingostomy, especially if the opposite tube has been removed previously or appears damaged.

It is often difficult in stable patients to differentiate between intra- and extrauterine pregnancy. In these situations the term 'pregnancy of unknown location' is often used. Such patients are followed up within an Early Pregnancy Assessment Unit (EPAU) setting with β-HCG monitoring and scans when necessary. As ectopic pregnancy is not ruled out in these patients, open access to an EPAU is necessary in case of increasing symptoms.

Placental abruption and placenta praevia

The patient is obese and it is possible that she has a concealed advanced pregnancy. Conditions associated with later pregnancy presenting with vaginal bleeding may be relevant to her.

She reports a period 8 weeks ago, so it is important to establish if this had been a normal period for her. As spotting does occur during pregnancy this could mean that she is advanced in a pregnancy, making the conditions of placental abruption, or placenta praevia more relevant.

Placental abruption refers to disruption of the placental attachment to the uterus by haemorrhage. Bleeding from the placenta occurs and the resultant haematoma formation causes further separation and compromise of the blood supply to the fetus. The severity of fetal distress depends on the degree of separation, but if it is complete or nearly complete, fetal death is inevitable unless immediate Caesarean section can be performed. Placental abruption is thought to occur in approximately 1% of all pregnancies worldwide (see Box 5.3). The associated perinatal mortality rate is around 15% and there is a significant associated maternal morbidity due to haemorrhage and coagulopathy.

Painful vaginal bleeding is the commonest presenting complaint. On examination a tender, tonically contracted uterus can be felt, often associated with fetal distress (see Figure 5.3).

Placenta praevia is an obstetric complication of the second and third trimesters and one of the main causes of vaginal bleeding. It occurs when the placenta covers the cervical os to varying degrees and can be described as total, partial or marginal (see Figure 5.4). It occurs in 0.5% of pregnancies and has a mortality rate of 0.03%, with most deaths due to haemorrhage and coagulopathy. The exact aetiology is unknown but risk factors include high parity, multiple pregnancy, advanced maternal age, and previous Caesarean section or miscarriage.

Sudden onset of bright red, painless vaginal bleeding during the third trimester is the most common presentation. The woman may be haemodynamically compromised but the uterus is soft and non-tender which is not the case in placental abruption. An initial bleed may be self limiting though recurrent and profuse bleeding are well recognised.

In most units low lying placentas are identified at the detailed anomaly scan between 19 and 23 weeks. If a patient with a low lying placenta is bleeding, vaginal examination including speculum examination should be avoided due to the risk of further bleeding.

Dysfunctional uterine bleeding

Dysfunctional uterine bleeding (DUB) is the most common cause of vaginal bleeding during reproductive years and is the most likely diagnosis in the patient if she is not pregnant. In most cases (90%) it is due to anovulatory cycles when the corpus luteum fails to form,

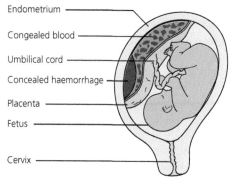

Endometrium

Congealed blood

Umbilical cord

Concealed haemorrhage

Placenta

Fetus

Cervix

Figure 5.3 Placental abruption.

resulting in a failure of cyclical progesterone secretion. The resulting unopposed oestrogens stimulate excess growth of the endometrium which eventually necroses and is shed. In ovulatory DUB prolonged progesterone secretion causes irregular shedding of the endometrium and spotting. This form is associated with polycystic ovary syndrome and other causes of altered hypothalamic function.

A normal menstrual cycle occurs every 21–35 days and lasts from 2–7 days. Average blood loss is 35–150 ml which represents up to eight soaked tampons or towels per day; usually no more than 2 days are heavy.

Menorrhagia is prolonged or excessive uterine bleeding occurring at regular intervals. Bleeding may also be irregular and/or more frequent than normal.

DUB is common and morbidity is related to the degree of blood loss which is rarely, but occasionally, severe enough to be life threatening. It can occur at any age but is most common at either end of the reproductive years. It is usually diagnosed when other causes of vaginal bleeding have been ruled out.

Women usually present following heavy or prolonged bleeding. It is important when taking the history to try to quantify the amount of blood loss by asking how many pads or tampons per day the woman is using, whether she is passing clots, or flooding. Similarly, symptoms and signs of anaemia should be looked for.

Prolonged periods are usually treated with oral progestagens such as norethisterone 5 mg three times a day to stop the bleeding. If the bleeding is heavy, tranexamic acid, 1 g four times a day may be helpful.

Local causes of vaginal bleeding

Infection (commonly *Chlamydia* and *Trichomonas*), cervical polyps or cervical erosions often present as post-coital bleeding or intermenstrual bleeding. Vaginal speculum examination usually reveals the cause. Triple swabs should be taken to investigate for infection.

Cervical cancer can present with similar symptoms and it is important that the cervix is visualised if bleeding is persistent.

Case history revisited

Given the differential diagnoses, ascertaining whether this woman is pregnant is important. Additional questions concerning the symptoms of pregnancy should be asked, e.g. nausea, morning sickness, breast tenderness, tiredness.

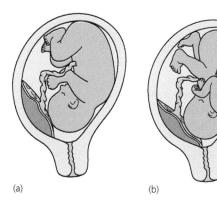

(a)   (b)   (c)

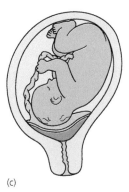

Figure 5.4 Placenta praevia. (a) Normal placenta. (b) Minor placenta praevia. (c) Major placenta praevia.

Examination

On examination she looks distressed, pale and cool. Vital signs are pulse 40 beats/ minute, blood pressure 86/40 mmHg, respiratory rate 22/minute. Her abdomen is not distended but she is tender suprapubically. Bowel sounds are normal. A pregnancy test is positive.

Question: Given the history and examination findings what is your principal working diagnosis?

Principal working diagnosis – Incomplete miscarriage with associated cervical shock

This woman is pregnant, has heavy vaginal bleeding, and is in shock with a bradycardia. Such findings strongly suggest that she has retained tissue in the os giving rise to cervical shock.

Management

The patient should be resuscitated with oxygen and intravenous fluid via two large bore, proximal cannulae.

The presence of a bradycardia should prompt examination of the cervix to remove any tissue in the os. Products of conception in the cervical os are easily removed with sponge forceps.

Once resuscitated the patient's condition should be discussed with the local EPAU and appropriate transfer or outpatient follow up arranged depending on levels of pain, bleeding and observations.

Patients should be immediately evaluated for haemodynamic stability, and fluid resuscitation initiated if required. Oxytocin may be required if bleeding is severe. In a rhesus-negative patient who is pregnant and bleeding *per vaginum*, rhesus (D) immune globulin should be administered if the pregnancy is 12 weeks or more, to prevent haemolytic disease of the newborn in future pregnancies.

Investigation of bleeding in early pregnancy is usually through an EPAU. Patients are seen by specialist nursing staff in an outpatient setting where ultrasound scans and blood investigations can be performed as necessary. These units reduce the need for patients to be admitted to hospital.

Outcome

This woman's condition dramatically improved once tissue was removed from her cervical os. She was allowed home after overnight observations and all her symptoms had settled when reviewed in the EPAU 2 days later.

Further reading

Knot A, Polmear A. *Practical General Practice: Guidelines for Effective Clinical Management*, Fourth Edition. Butterworth-Heinemann, Oxford, 2004.

Simon C, Everitt H, Kendrick T. *Oxford Handbook of General Practice*, Second Edition. Oxford University Press, Oxford, 2002.

Wyatt JP, Illingworth R, Graham C *et al. Oxford Handbook of Emergency Medicine*, Third Edition. Oxford University Press, Oxford, 2006.

CHAPTER 6

Transient Weakness

Carole Gavin

CASE HISTORY

A 70-year-old woman presents after suddenly developing a left-sided facial weakness and some clumsiness of her left hand 40 minutes previously. Her symptoms have improved but her face still feels heavy. She is a diabetic prescribed gliclazide and has recently begun medication for hypertension. She had a mastectomy for breast cancer 6 years ago and has recently been discharged from follow up. She has smoked 20 cigarettes a day for the past 40 years. Over the past few weeks she has had intermittent frontal headache and occasional nausea following a minor head injury but otherwise has felt well. She lives alone and is normally fully independent.

Table 6.1 Causes of transient neurology.

Central nervous system	Minor stroke/TIA
	Hemiplegic migraine
	Todd's paresis
	Subdural haematoma
	Brain tumour
	Cerebral abscess
Peripheral nervous system	Peripheral neuropathy
	Neuropraxia
	Bell's palsy
Metabolic/miscellaneous	Hypoglycaemia
	Hypokalaemia
	Hypocalcaemia
	Decompression sickness ('the bends')
	Hysteria

Question: What differential diagnosis would you consider from the history?

There are various causes of transient neurological symptoms (see Table 6.1) which can be divided into conditions affecting the central nervous system, conditions affecting the peripheral nervous system and those due to metabolic abnormalities.

Hypoglycaemia

The patient is diabetic, on gliclazide and is therefore prone to hypoglycaemia. Hypoglycaemia is an important cause of neurological symptoms and signs and all patients should have blood glucose measured at the bedside. It is well recognised that patients with apparently dense strokes dramatically improve and return to normal when their hypoglycaemia is treated.

Transient ischaemic attack (TIA)/minor stroke

This patient has a number of risk factors for cerebrovascular disease. Stroke is the commonest cause of a unilateral motor and/or sensory deficit. Traditionally a TIA was defined as a sudden, focal neurological deficit lasting for less than 24 hours, presumed to be of vascular origin, and confined to an area of the brain or eye perfused by a specific artery. However, it is now known that transient neurological symptoms may be associated with cerebral infarction

on brain imaging and that in reality most TIAs resolve within 1 hour. A new definition has therefore been proposed that TIA is a brief episode of neurological dysfunction caused by focal brain or retinal ischemia, with clinical symptoms typically lasting less than 1 hour, and without evidence of acute infarction. Stroke and TIA are therefore best thought of as two ends of the spectrum of acute brain ischaemia. Risk factors for both are the same and include hypertension, hyperlipidaemia, smoking, diabetes and atrial fibrillation. Typical symptoms include hemiparesis, hemiparesthesia, dysarthria, dysphasia, diplopia, circumoral numbness, imbalance, and monocular blindness depending on the vascular territory involved. The ROSIER scale (Recognition of Stroke in the Emergency Room) (see Figure 6.1) is a useful stroke recognition tool for staff seeing the patient in the acute phase. When making a diagnosis of TIA it is important to establish that the symptoms were focal, came on suddenly and were maximal at onset. Another key point is that symptoms of TIA are usually 'negative', e.g. loss of power, loss of sensation, loss of vision, whilst 'positive' symptoms, e.g. pins and needles, abnormal movements suggest an alternative diagnosis.

Subdural haematoma

This woman has had a head injury within the past few weeks so the possibility of a subdural haematoma must be considered. These arise in the potential space between the dura and arachnoid, often from ruptured bridging veins. The space enlarges as the brain atrophies and so subdural haematomas are more common in the elderly. Symptoms are often vague and may develop slowly

ABC of Emergency Differential Diagnosis. Edited by F. Morris and A. Fletcher. © 2009 Blackwell Publishing, ISBN: 978-1-4051-7063-5.

A&E STROKE RECOGNITION INSTRUMENT

Date/Time of symptom onset ....

GCS E = ☐ M = ☐ V = ☐   BP ....../......   *BM...............

*If BM < 3.5 mmol/l treat urgently and reassess once blood glucose normal

Has there been loss of consciousness or syncope?   Y(−1) ☐ N(0) ☐

Has there been seizure activity?   Y(−1) ☐ N(0) ☐

Is there a <u>NEW ACUTE</u> onset (or on awakening from sleep)

Asymmetric facial weakness	Y(+1) ☐	N(0) ☐
Asymmetric grip weakness	Y(+1) ☐	N(0) ☐
Asymmetric arm weakness	Y(+1) ☐	N(0) ☐
Asymmetric leg weakness	Y(+1) ☐	N(0) ☐
Speech disturbance	Y(+1) ☐	N(0) ☐
Visual field defect	Y(+1) ☐	N(0) ☐

*Total Score.......... (−2 to +6)

Provisional diagnosis

☐ Stroke

☐ Non-stroke (specify)................................

*stroke is unlikely but not completely excluded if total scores ≤ 0

Figure 6.1 ROSIER Scale proforma.

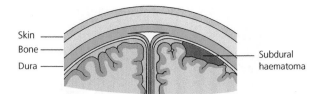

Figure 6.2 Illustration of a subdural haematoma.

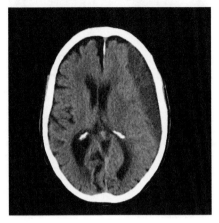

Figure 6.3 Subdural haematoma.

with gradual deterioration or fluctuation in conscious level. Focal symptoms may develop due to mass effect on the brain tissue (see Figures 6.2 and 6.3).

Hemiplegic migraine

Migraine may be associated with sensory, motor or aphasic aura. Hemiplegic migraine is characterised by unilateral sensory and/or motor signs. Sensory auras occur more frequently than motor auras and usually affect the hand and arm. In over 90% of cases the aura precedes the onset of headache. The diagnosis should be considered in patients who have a previous history of hemiplegic migraine, but if the aura has lasted for longer than an hour neuroimaging may be required to exclude migrainous infarction. The diagnosis of hemiplegic migraine is one of exclusion if the patient has no previous history of migraine, as in the case of this woman, or if the history differs from their usual migraine symptoms.

Todd's paresis

Todd's paresis (also called post-ictal paresis), is a transient neurological deficit following an epileptic seizure. As the name implies, the classical deficit is weakness of a hand, arm or leg that appears following focal motor seizure activity. The neurological signs are unilateral and range in duration from seconds to over 20 minutes. The diagnosis may be apparent from the history if the focal deficit follows a witnessed fit and should be considered in a patient with a history of epilepsy. A small proportion of patients with a stroke

may present with a fit so if the neurological symptoms persist for longer than an hour neuroimaging should be performed.

Brain tumour

This patient has a history of breast cancer and may have a cerebral metastasis. Patients with primary or metastatic brain tumours may present with transient focal neurological symptoms. Suspicion should be raised if the neurological deficit does not fit with a single vascular territory as would be the case with a stroke or TIA, and if there are any 'positive' as opposed to 'negative' symptoms. The patient should be asked about other symptoms such as headache, cognitive impairment, or nausea and vomiting that may indicate raised intracranial pressure. The diagnosis is usually made by CT or MRI scan.

Other causes of transient weakness not suggested by the history

Bell's palsy

Bell's palsy is defined as an acute peripheral facial nerve palsy of unknown cause, although herpes simplex viral activation has become widely accepted as the likely cause in the majority of cases. Patients typically present with unilateral facial weakness which may be associated with an inability to close the eye and difficulty eating or speaking due to facial weakness (see Figure 6.4). Patients often think that their symptoms are due to a stroke and it may be misdiagnosed as such by inexperienced junior doctors. Its differentiation from a central (upper motor neurone) condition such as a stroke is suggested by an inability to elevate the brow as this area receives bilateral innervation. However, a partial peripheral lesion that spares the temporal branch to the frontalis will result in the patient still being able to wrinkle the forehead. The course tends to be progressive

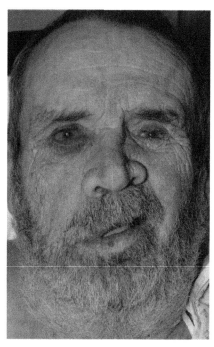

Figure 6.4 Right sided Bell's palsy.

over several weeks, usually resolving to at least some degree within 6 months. The auditory meatus should be examined for the presence of herpetic vesicles which may support the diagnosis. Initial management consists of eye care, steroids and antiviral treatment. Follow up should be arranged as further investigation is warranted if the symptoms do not resolve. In this woman the clumsiness in her hand excludes Bell's palsy as a cause of her symptoms.

Peripheral neuropathy

Focal motor and/or sensory deficit may arise as a result of a peripheral nerve palsy or mononeuropathy. Sudden onset of motor weakness, e.g. foot drop, due to peripheral neuropathy may be thought to be a stroke by the patient or an unwary clinician. Making the diagnosis may be difficult as it depends on recognising that the neurological deficit is confined to the distribution of a single nerve, and requires good knowledge of peripheral nerve anatomy and of the motor and sensory territories of each nerve. Common causes include trauma, external compression, internal compression, e.g. median nerve entrapment in the carpal tunnel, or intrinsic lesions to the nerve, e.g. arising as a focal manifestation of a more generalised process such as vasculitis. Common nerves involved are shown in Table 6.2. Symptoms may be transient, e.g. external compression of the nerve following an episode of sleep, making the diagnosis even more difficult if the symptoms have resolved by the time the patient is seen. In the case of this patient she had symptoms in two different nerve territories thus making the diagnosis unlikely.

Metabolic disturbance

Several metabolic abnormalities may cause neurological symptoms. Hypocalcaemia may cause transient parasthesia especially of the peripheries. It may be accompanied by a history of hyperventilation and other symptoms such as tetany or carpopedal spasm.

Table 6.2 Common peripheral neuropathies.

Nerve	Symptoms/signs
Radial nerve	Wrist drop 'Saturday night palsy'
Ulnar	Paraesthesia ring and little fingers Reduced power of grip
Median	Carpal tunnel syndrome: paraesthesia of thumb, index and middle fingers
Common peroneal	Foot drop Paraesthesia dorsum of foot
Lumbosacral radiculopathies:	
L5	Decreased foot dorsiflexion, inversion and eversion
L2–4	Weakness of hip flexion, knee extension and leg abduction Reduced sensation anterior thigh to medial aspect of shin

Hypokalemia or hyperkalaemia may cause episodes of severe muscle weakness (periodic paralysis). It may be associated with cardiac arrhythmias and an ECG should be performed urgently pending blood results.

Symptoms resulting from metabolic abnormalities tend to be generalised rather than focal and therefore are unlikely to be the cause of this woman's problem.

Decompression sickness

Decompression sickness may cause paraesthesia or weakness due to involvement of the spinal cord. It may be associated with joint pains, rash and delirium and the diagnosis is usually obvious from the history. Consider it in people returning from holiday who may have been diving.

Case history revisited

This woman tells you that prior to going to sleep she felt perfectly well. She has never experienced anything like this before and does not have any history of migraine or epilepsy. Her occasional headaches usually occur at the end of the day and are completely relieved by paracetamol. Her daughter, who dialled 999, tells you that when her mother rang her to tell her she was unwell she thought her mother had been drinking as her speech seemed very slurred and she was slightly confused. She was very worried as her mother rarely drinks. She now appears to be back to her normal self and thinks the symptoms lasted about 90 minutes in total.

Examination

On clinical examination there is no obvious focal neurological deficit and speech and cognition are normal. Blood pressure is 140/70 mmHg and heart rate is 90 beats/minute. Blood glucose is 7.5 mmol/l. Respiratory and gastrointestinal examination is normal. There is no evidence of Bell's palsy and ear, nose and throat examination is normal. An ECG confirms sinus rhythmn.

Question: Given the history and examination findings what is your principal working diagnosis?

Principal working diagnosis – TIA

The combination of transient left-sided face and hand weakness associated with speech disturbance is compatible with a transient ischaemic attack. This woman has a number of risk factors including hypertension, smoking and diabetes. Patients who have had a TIA have up to a 20% risk of stroke in the first month with the risk being greatest in the first 72 hours. The key points in the acute management of such patients is therefore to identify and address any modifiable risk factors (see Table 6.3), to initiate antiplatelet treatment if appropriate, and to identify those patients at greatest risk in order to prioritise investigation and referral for definitive management such as carotid endarterectomy.

The ABCD2 score is a validated prognostic score (see Tables 6.4 and 6.5) that has been proposed in order to identify those patients at greatest risk of stroke who are most likely to benefit from early intervention.

Table 6.3 Risk factors for stroke.

Risk factor	Investigation
Hypertension	Blood pressure measurement
Diabetes mellitis	Blood sugar
Hyperlipidaemia	Lipid profile
Atrial fibrillation	ECG
Carotid artery stenosis	Carotid Doppler ultrasound

Table 6.4 ABCD2 score.

ABCD2 score variable	
Choose appropriate single score from each section	
Age	
<60 years	0
60 years or above	1
Blood pressure	
SBP >140 mmHg *or* DBP >90 mmHg	1
BP below these levels	0
Clinical features	
Any unilateral weakness (face/hand/arm/leg)	2
Speech disturbance (without motor weakness)	1
Other weakness	0
Duration of symptoms	
>60 minutes	2
10–59 minutes	1
<10 minutes	0
Diabetic	
Yes	1
No	0

Table 6.5 Risk stratification by ABCD2 score.

ABCD2 score	Risk category	Stroke risk
0	Low	1% at 2 days
1		1.2% at 7 days
2		3.1% at 90 days
3		
4	Moderate	4.1% at 2 days
5		5.9% at 7 days
		9.8% at 90 days
6	High	8.1% at 2 days
7		11.7% at 7 days
		17.8% at 90 days

Outcome

This lady had an ABCD2 score of 5. Full blood count, biochemical profile and random lipid profile were all normal. A CT scan of the brain was normal. She was reviewed by the acute stroke team who arranged for carotid Doppler ultrasound to be performed in 2 days time as an outpatient. She was given a 300 mg stat dose of aspirin and discharged on 75 mg aspirin daily pending review in the TIA clinic in 5 days time. She was advised to stop smoking and to return to the hospital immediately in the event of any further symptoms.

Further reading

Patten JP. *Neurological Differential Diagnosis*. Springer-Verlag, Berlin, 1995.

Ramrakha P, Moore K. *Oxford Handbook of Acute Medicine*, Second Edition. Oxford University Press, Oxford, 2004.

Simon C, Everitt H, Kendrick T. *Oxford Handbook of General Practice*, Second Edition. Oxford University Press, Oxford, 2002.

Tintinalli J, Kelen G, Stapczynski S, *et al. Emergency Medicine: A Comprehensive Study Guide*, Sixth Edition. McGraw-Hill, New York, 2003.

Wyatt JP, Illingworth R, Graham C, *et al. Oxford Handbook of Emergency Medicine*, Third Edition. Oxford University Press, Oxford, 2006.

CHAPTER 7

Abdominal Pain – Epigastric

Duncan Drury

CASE HISTORY

A 44-year-old man presents with upper abdominal pain. He gives a history of intermittent episodes of upper abdominal pain for which he has taken both ibuprofen and antacids in the past. On the morning of presentation he was working in the garden, chopping down trees. He had been experiencing some abdominal pain for the last few days but it was bothering him more than normal. He had just enjoyed a typical Sunday lunch with his wife and had three glasses of wine, when he suddenly developed epigastric pain which was much more severe than earlier. The pain was of such intensity that he felt short of breath, nauseated and started sweating. In the past he had suffered from hypertension for which he is taking amlodipine. He was recently prescribed ramipril to improve his blood pressure control, along with aspirin 75 mg daily. He is an ex-smoker having given up 6 months ago. He also admits to being a moderate drinker since he was made redundant from his job as an office manager 4 months ago. He has no other significant past medical or surgical history.

Question: What differential diagnosis would you consider from the history?

Gallstones

The prevalence of gallstones in the UK is estimated to be 10–20% and approximately 20% of these remain asymptomatic. They are composed of cholesterol, bile pigments or a combination of both. They are usually diagnosed on an ultrasound scan but are occasionally visible on a plain abdominal X-ray (see Figure 7.1). Gallstones may present with acute cholecystitis due to obstruction of Hartman's pouch or cystic duct culminating in inflammation of the gallbladder and typically right upper quadrant or epigastric pain that may radiate to the back or shoulder tip. It is frequently associated with nausea and vomiting. Such patients often have a fever, tachycardia and right upper quadrant tenderness and guarding. Pain on inspiration and on palpation of the right upper quadrant (Murphy's sign) is typical of acute cholecystitis.

Gallstones may also present with biliary colic (often significant abdominal pain but minimal/mild abdominal tenderness). Biliary

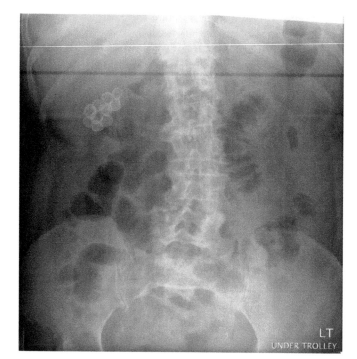

Figure 7.1 Gallstones on plain X-ray.

colic is due to smooth muscle contraction of either the cystic duct or common bile duct in an attempt to clear a gallstone and may be associated with abnormal liver function tests if the stone is causing significant duct obstruction.

Gastritis/duodenitis/peptic ulcer

Inflammation of the stomach/duodenum may range from superficial erosions in the mucosal lining to ulceration which is usually larger and deeper. The commonest risk factors include non-steroidal anti-inflammatory drug (NSAID) use, aspirin, alcohol, *Helicobacter pylori* and biliary reflux. Duodenal ulcers are significantly more common than gastric ulcers and are more commonly associated with *H. pylori* than gastric ulcers. Symptoms may vary from asymptomatic to indigestion, vomiting and bleeding. There is a poor correlation between intensity of symptoms and endoscopic severity of the disease. Treatment is with proton pump inhibitors coupled with *H. Pylori* eradication if found to be present.

ABC of Emergency Differential Diagnosis. Edited by F. Morris and A. Fletcher. © 2009 Blackwell Publishing, ISBN: 978-1-4051-7063-5.

Perforated peptic ulcer disease

Untreated, a peptic ulcer may progress to perforation resulting in initially localised peritonitis, subsequently becoming generalised if the condition is not treated. Typically a patient has symptoms associated with gastritis (see above) but subsequent perforation results in a sudden increase in upper abdominal pain that may radiate through to the back. Nausea is fairly common as are findings of tachycardia, dehydration and low grade pyrexia. On examination, there is significant epigastric tenderness with signs of either localised or generalised peritonism (guarding, rigidity, rebound and percussion tenderness). Bowel sounds are often absent reflecting an ileus that often ensues.

Pancreatitis

Acute pancreatitis is characterised by severe epigastric pain typically radiating through to the back. It is often associated with nausea and vomiting. There are many causes of pancreatitis (see Box 7.1), but the vast majority of cases in the UK are due to gallstones and alcohol. The patient with mild pancreatitis may have very few signs or may have shock, pyrexia, generalised abdominal tenderness and guarding with abdominal wall discolouration (peri-umbilical – Cullen's sign, flanks – Grey Turner's sign) with severe necrotising pancreatitis. Diagnosis is confirmed either biochemically (serum amylase greater than four times the upper limit of the laboratory reference range), or radiologically. Investigations include ultrasound, contrast-enhanced CT and MRI, and are used to establish the cause and assess the severity and complications.

Box 7.1 **Causes of acute pancreatitis**

G	Gallstones
E	Ethanol
T	Trauma
S	Steroids
M	Mumps
A	Autoimmune (e.g. polyarteritis nodosa)
S	Scorpion bites
H	Hyperlipidaemia, hypercalcaemia, hypothermia
E	ERCP (endoscopic retrograde cholangiopancreatography)
D	Drugs (e.g. azathioprine, mercaptopurine)

Musculoskeletal

A pain of musculoskeletal origin should be suspected if the patient gives a history of trauma or unaccustomed exertion prior to the development of pain. In the event of a significant mechanism of injury, damage to internal solid organs (particularly blunt trauma), or damage to the viscera (particularly with rapid deceleration forces), should always be considered and actively ruled out. A diagnosis of musculoskeletal pain would only be made with an appropriate history coupled with the absence of any other abnormalities (i.e. normal temperature, blood pressure and pulse rate backed up by normal biochemical, haematological and radiological investigations).

Myocardial infarction

This would typically present with severe chest pain that often occurs at rest associated with nausea, vomiting, sweating and breathlessness, and may radiate to the neck or arms. However, atypical presentations of myocardial infarction are well recognised and the pain may be experienced exclusively in the epigastrium. Consequently, ischaemic heart disease should always be considered in the differential diagnosis of any at risk patient presenting with epigastric pain (see Figure 7.2).

Other causes of epigastric abdominal pain not suggested by the history

Leaking abdominal aortic aneurysm (AAA)

An aneurysm is a focal dilatation of an artery to more than 50% of that of the normal adjacent vessel. The prevalence of AAA is estimated to be 7–8% of men aged 65 years and older and is therefore unlikely in a man aged 44.

A ruptured aneurysm should always be considered in a patient with sudden onset severe abdominal pain radiating to the back, associated with circulatory collapse. Rupture into the retroperitoneal space is initially contained by the resultant hypotension and tamponading effect of bleeding into a fixed space. This situation must be rapidly diagnosed to provide an opportunity for emergency life-saving vascular intervention. Free intraperitoneal rupture or subsequent rupture of a retroperitoneal bleed is invariably fatal.

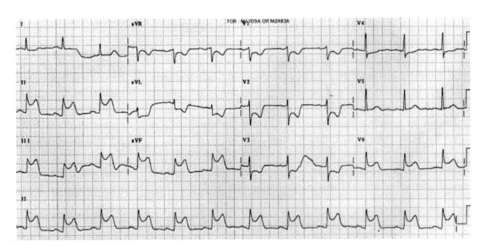

Figure 7.2 Infero-lateral myocardial infarction.

Other uncommon causes are contained in Box 7.2

> **Box 7.2 Uncommon causes of upper abdominal pain**
>
> - Pulmonary embolism
> - Basal pneumonia (see Figure 7.3)
> - Ischaemic bowel
> - Dissecting aortic aneurysm
> - Addison's disease
> - Hypercalcaemia
> - Renal colic

> **Box 7.3 Blood test results**
>
> - FBC – Hb 14.6, WCC 15.0, Plt 315
> - U+Es – Na$^+$ 141, K$^+$ 3.9, Urea 8.0, Creatinine 122
> - LFTs – Normal
> - Amylase – 170 (ref. range 70–140)
> - Glucose – 6.2
> - Calcium (corrected) – 2.46
> - Cardiac markers (performed at 12 h) – normal

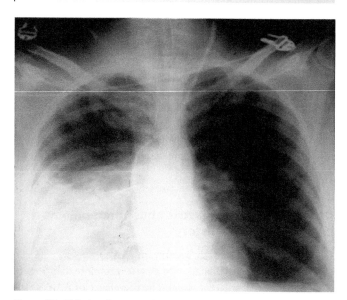

Figure 7.3 Right basal pneumonia.

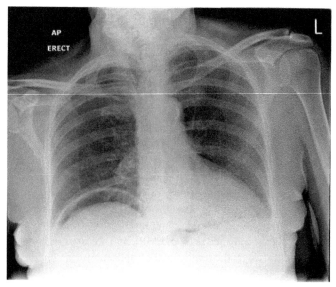

Figure 7.4 Erect chest X-ray.

Case history revisited

This patient's history is quite non-specific and a number of diagnoses are quite plausible. A musculoskeletal cause for the pain whilst possible would be unlikely given his relative inactivity at the time of deterioration. He does have a number of risk factors for cardiovascular diseases (male gender, increasing age, hypertension, ex-smoker) and gastrointestinal diseases (alcohol intake, aspirin, NSAIDs and stress from recent unemployment).

Examination

In order to determine the diagnosis in this patient a thorough physical examination and further investigations are required.

On examination, he is apyrexial with a blood pressure of 140/80 mmHg and is tachycardic at 110 beats/min. His respiratory rate is 22 breaths/minute and his oxygen saturation is 97% on air. He is still complaining of pain in his abdomen.

Examination of his cardiorespiratory system is unremarkable other than the tachycardia and tachypnoea.

Examination of his abdomen demonstrates marked epigastric tenderness with generalised rigidity, guarding and rebound tenderness. His bowel sounds are absent. No masses were felt.

An ECG revealed sinus tachycardia but was otherwise normal. His blood test results are seen in Box 7.3. His chest X-ray is seen in Figure 7.4.

Question: Given the history, examination findings and investigations what is your principal working diagnosis?

Principal working diagnosis – perforated peptic ulcer

The clinical findings are those of peritonitis.

His history contains several risk factors for peptic ulcer disease: NSAID usage, alcohol usage and stress. His symptoms have persisted for some time and with the sudden onset of worsening pain, his rigid abdomen and free air under the diaphragm all suggest perforation of an underlying peptic ulcer.

Management

He requires rehydration with intravenous fluids to restore his circulatory volume. A combination of vomiting and sequestration of fluid within the gastrointestinal tract (third space loss) almost always results in dehydration at presentation that needs correcting prior to surgical intervention. He requires a urinary catheter to ensure good urine output and to confirm he is adequately fluid resuscitated. In addition, he should be given broad spectrum intravenous antibiotics (cefuroxime and metronidazole). The surgical team should review him and consideration given to an urgent laparotomy. This man was resuscitated and taken to theatre, where he underwent emergency surgery. This confirmed a perforated pre-pyloric gastric ulcer. He underwent thorough peritoneal lavage and oversewing of his ulcer.

Outcome

Post-operatively he made an uneventful recovery and was treated with a proton pump inhibitor. A course of *H. pylori* eradication therapy was undertaken as he was found to have a positive serology. Upon discharge he underwent a check endoscopy to confirm both healing of the ulcer and successful eradication of *H. pylori*.

Further reading

Knot A, Polmear A. *Practical General Practice: Guidelines for Effective Clinical Management*, Fourth Edition. Butterworth-Heinemann, Oxford, 2004.

Simon C, Everitt H, Kendrick T. *Oxford Handbook of General Practice*, Second Edition. Oxford University Press, Oxford, 2002.

Tintinalli J, Kelen G, Stapczynski S, *et al. Emergency Medicine: A Comprehensive Study Guide*. Sixth Edition. McGraw-Hill, New York, 2003.

Wyatt JP, Illingworth R, Graham C, *et al. Oxford Handbook of Emergency Medicine*, Third Edition. Oxford University Press, Oxford, 2006.

CHAPTER 8

Acute Headache

Tom Locker

Question: What differential diagnosis would you consider from the history?

Subarachnoid haemorrhage

Sudden, severe, explosive headaches (thunderclap) may be the result of a number of different conditions (see Box 8.1).

Only 12% of such patients will have a subarachnoid haemorrhage (SAH) although up to two-thirds of patients presenting to hospital with this type of headache, investigated as an inpatient, have a serious underlying disorder.

The majority of SAHs (see Figure 8.1) result from rupture of cerebral artery aneurysms and usually occur in people aged between 40 and 60.

The key feature of the headache in SAH is the sudden onset rather than the severity of headache. The headache is frequently described as 'the worst ever' although occasionally it may be moderate or mild in severity. The onset of headache in SAH may be associated with activities that cause a transient increase in blood pressure such as straining, lifting heavy objects, etc.

The site of the headache is variable and therefore not a useful guide to diagnosis. Fronto-temporal headaches as well as the 'classical' occipital headache are well recognised in SAH.

Given these features, any patient presenting with a sudden onset of severe headache should be investigated further to rule out a subarachnoid haemorrhage. Migraine is an unsafe diagnosis in such patients unless there is a clear history of multiple previous episodes of the same headache.

Box 8.1 **Causes of thunderclap headache**

- Subarachnoid haemorrhage
- Intracerebral haemorrhage
- Venous sinus thrombosis
- Meningitis
- Encephalitis
- Migraine
- Cough headache
- Coital headache
- Pituitary apoplexy
- Spontaneous intracranial hypotension

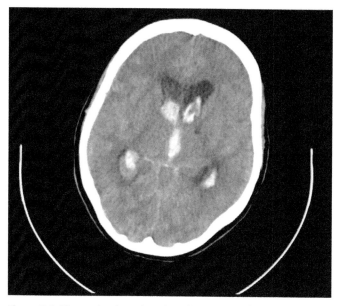

Figure 8.1 CT scan showing subarachnoid haemorrhage with bleeding into the ventricles.

Clinical examination may reveal a decreased conscious level, signs of meningeal irritation (see Table 8.1) or focal neurological abnormalities. However, examination may be entirely normal.

Migraine

Migraine affects up to 15% of adults in North America and Western Europe. It typically lasts between 4 and 72 hours unless successfully terminated by drug treatment. There are two main types

ABC of Emergency Differential Diagnosis. Edited by F. Morris and A. Fletcher. © 2009 Blackwell Publishing, ISBN: 978-1-4051-7063-5.

Table 8.1 Signs of meningeal irritation.

Neck stiffness	With the patient supine the head is held by the examiner. The neck is passively flexed and the amount of resistance noted. The sign is positive when there is objective stiffness, not when the patient reports a subjective feeling of stiffness.
	Painful inflammatory conditions of the pharynx, such as tonsillitis or quinsy may result in a false positive finding.
Brudzinski's sign	In Brudzinski's sign flexion of the hips and knees occurring in response to passive flexion of the neck indicates meningeal irritation.
Kernig's sign	With the patient supine the hip and knee are passively flexed to 90 degrees. The knee is then passively extended. The sign is positive when there is resistance to extension.
	This test usefully distinguishes meningeal irritation from the local cause of neck stiffness described above.

Box 8.2 **Features of migraine**

The headache has at least two of the following features:
- unilateral location
- pulsating quality
- moderate or severe intensity
- aggravation by physical activity
At least one of the following occur during the headache:
- nausea and/or vomiting
- Photophobia or phonophobia

---

of migraine: without aura and with aura. The characteristics of migraine without aura are shown in Box 8.2.

In migraine with aura the patient may experience visual symptoms, such as lines in the vision or loss of vision, sensory symptoms, or dysphasia. The aura lasts between 5 and 60 minutes and is followed within an hour by a headache fulfilling the criteria in Box 8.2.

Some patients are able to identify particular triggers for their migraine. These may include alcohol, certain foods, alterations in sleep pattern or menstruation.

Caution should be exercised in attributing focal neurological abnormalities, e.g. dysphasia or weakness to migraine, unless the patient has previously experienced a number of similar episodes from which they have recovered. In the acute setting migraine is a diagnosis of exclusion.

Meningitis

The headache in meningitis is not typically of sudden onset but given the dangers of missing the diagnosis it is a condition that should always be considered in the differential diagnosis of a patient presenting with a severe headache.

Meningitis may result from bacterial, viral, or less commonly fungal or tuberculous infection. The diagnosis is suggested by the complaint of a headache in association with fever and neck stiffness, which is found in two-thirds of patients with bacterial meningitis. In addition, signs of meningeal irritation (see Table 8.1) should also be sought but may be absent early in the course of the illness. A high index of suspicion therefore needs to be maintained, particularly in the elderly or immunocompromised patient.

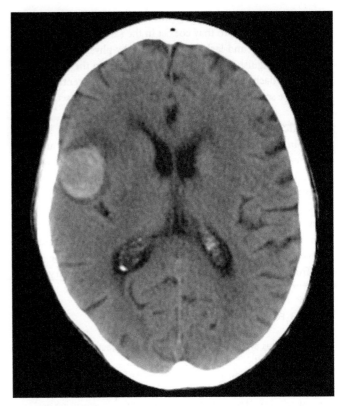

Figure 8.2 CT scan of an intracerebral metastatic neoplasm.

In contrast, the absence of fever, neck stiffness and change in mental state reliably excludes meningitis.

Space-occupying lesions

It is uncommon for intracranial mass lesions to present with sudden severe headache. Such lesions only cause pain once they are large enough to cause traction on intracranial vessels or invade sensitive structures such as the dura. As a result, such lesions will often present with other features before headache becomes prominent.

The headache caused by space-occupying lesions is usually the result of raised intracranial pressure. Typically this headache will be of gradual onset, progressively severe, worse in the morning, and aggravated by activities which raise intracranial pressure, for example coughing or straining.

A careful neurological examination may reveal subtle abnormalities of which the patient is unaware. The presence of papilloedema supports the diagnosis but its absence does not rule it out.

Sudden onset of headache may occur in a patient with a space-occupying lesion if there is haemorrhage into a tumour (see Figure 8.2).

Other causes of headache not suggested by the history

Tension headache

It is estimated that 80% of people will experience a tension headache at some time during their life. In contrast to migraine, the headache may last up to 7 days.

The key features of tension headache are shown in Box 8.3 and these headaches tend to be precipitated by stress.

Differentiating between migraine and tension headaches can be difficult and the two may coexist in the same patient. The non-pulsating quality and lack of aggravation by physical activity may usefully distinguish between the two. However, in the acute setting tension headache is not usually included in the differential diagnosis of acute severe headache as it is rarely of sudden onset.

Systemic illness

Severe infections such as pneumonia and pyelonephritis are a frequent cause of headache. Diagnosis in such patients is rarely difficult. As the headache is not of sudden onset, a careful history and examination will identify the cause.

Dental and ENT disease

Pain in the head or face is a key feature in many dental and ENT problems, e.g. sinusitis. Although the diagnosis may be apparent from the history, inspection of the mouth, pharynx and

> **Box 8.3 Features of tension headache**
>
> Headache has at least two of the following characteristics:
> - bilateral location
> - pressing/tightening (non-pulsating) quality
> - mild or moderate intensity
> - not aggravated by routine physical activity such as walking or climbing stairs
>
> And both of the following:
> - no nausea or vomiting (anorexia may occur)
> - no more than one of photophobia or phonophobia

tympanic membranes is required to exclude these as possible sources of pain.

Temporal arteritis

Temporal arteritis typically presents with gradual onset of a constant band-like headache and tenderness over the temporal arteries. It may also be associated with visual loss. Typically, patients will be over 55 years of age and feel generally unwell. The erythrocyte sedimentation rate is usually markedly raised. Urgent treatment with corticosteroids reduces the risk of visual loss.

Case history revisited

The history outlined by this woman suggests a number of possible diagnoses. The patient has a history of migraine, but this headache is clearly different to her usual migraine headache, so this is an unlikely cause. The history of breast cancer raises the possibility of a cerebral metastasis. Given the sudden onset of the headache and its severity, haemorrhage into a metastasis or into the subarachnoid space should be considered.

Her history of fever preceding the headache suggests that meningitis should be considered although the sudden onset of the headache makes this diagnosis less likely.

Examination

On examination the patient's observations are normal. Her temperature is 36.5°C, blood pressure 107/60 mmHg and pulse rate 90 beats/minute.

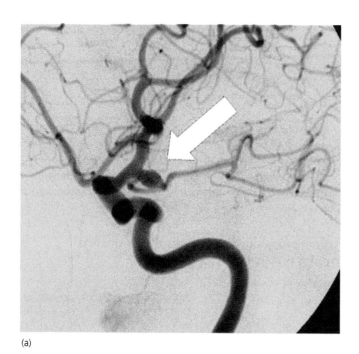

(a)

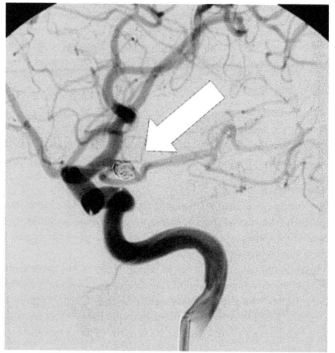

(b)

Figure 8.3 Intracranial aneurysm before (a) and after coiling (b).

Her neck was stiff but there is no other abnormality on neurological examination. Examination of the fundi and tympanic membranes is normal and there is no rash.

Question: Given the history and examination findings what is your principal working diagnosis?

Principal working diagnosis – subarachnoid haemorrhage

Management

The sudden onset of headache and the finding of neck stiffness suggest subarachnoid haemorrhage is the cause of her symptoms.

The next step will be to obtain a CT scan. In patients with subarachnoid haemorrhage this will be abnormal in around 95% of cases if the scan is performed within the first 24 hours, but only in 50% 1 week after onset of the headache. CT should also reliably exclude the possibility of a space-occupying lesion.

If the CT scan is normal a lumbar puncture should be performed. When investigating possible subarachnoid haemorrhage this should be delayed until 12 hours after onset of the headache, when its sensitivity will be maximal. If subarachnoid haemorrhage is not found, examination of the cerebrospinal fluid (CSF) should also identify cases of meningitis. In addition, the measurement of CSF pressure may also identify some uncommon diagnoses that might otherwise be missed, such as venous sinus thrombosis or spontaneous intracranial hypotension.

Outcome

The patient underwent a CT scan which demonstrated a subarachnoid haemorrhage (see Figure 8.3a). She was referred urgently to a neurosurgeon for further treatment. The causative aneurysm was subsequently coiled (see Figure 8.3b).

Further reading

Dowson AJ. *Your Questions Answered: Migraine and Other Headaches*. Churchill Livingstone, Edinburgh, 2003.

Lance JW, Goadsby PJ. *Mechanism and Management of Headache*, Seventh Edition. Elsevier, New York, 2005.

CHAPTER 9

Acutely Painful Joint

Rachel Tattersall

Question: What differential diagnosis would you consider from the history?

There are many possible causes of an acutely inflamed joint. Although the history must be comprehensive, key points are shown in Box 9.1. Physical examination should be comprehensive, and locomotor examination should start with the 'GALS' (Gait, Arms, Legs, Spine) screen. This is a quick and easy to perform screen of all the joints thereby identifying abnormal joints for closer examination and ensuring undeclared joint abnormalities do not go unnoticed. Once an abnormal joint is identified its appearance

Box 9.1 **Key history points in the patient with an acutely inflamed joint**

- Previous joint problems/other current joint problems
- Recent illness (gastric upset, sexually acquired infection)
- Exposure to infection such as drug misuse or dental work
- Skin rash
- Trauma/penetrating injury
- Alcohol intake/family history of gout/dietary history/hypertension
- Job/recent travel/pets
- Risk factors for HIV

ABC of Emergency Differential Diagnosis. Edited by F. Morris and A. Fletcher.
© 2009 Blackwell Publishing, ISBN: 978-1-4051-7063-5.

should be documented and then palpated to elicit warmth, tenderness and swelling. The range of movement should then be assessed. If in doubt – look, feel, move!

Septic arthritis

Patients with a short history of a hot, swollen and tender joint (or joints) with restriction of movement should be considered to have septic arthritis until proven otherwise. Septic arthritis is a medical emergency because untreated, joint destruction and systemic sepsis may follow. In adults, septic arthritis is usually monoarticular but polyarticular presentations are possible. Examination signs may include features of systemic infection such as fever, rashes, or even septic shock. Septic arthritis is usually very painful and any movement of the infected joint is often agonising.

Bacterial invasion of the synovial space most commonly follows haematogenous spread and the commonest infecting organism is *Staphylococcus aureus*. Direct innoculation of bacteria to the joint is also possible and a history of local trauma or penetrating injury should always be sought. Within 48 hours of bacterial invasion of the synovial space there is dramatic neutrophil infiltration, vascular congestion and cellular proliferation leading to purulent effusion and the cytokine-induced release of proteolytic enzymes. In as little as 10 days cartilage and bone destruction develop, so in making the diagnosis time is of the essence. The history should focus on risk factors for septic arthritis. These are the extremes of the age spectrum, chronic disease such as diabetes mellitus and human immunodeficiency virus (HIV) infection, prosthetic joints, pre-existing inflammatory arthritis and procedures leading to bacteraemia such as dental treatment or injecting drug use. Immunocompromise also predisposes to infection, and a full medication history is important.

Gonococcal arthritis results from haematogenous spread of *Neisseria* gonococcus from primary sexually acquired mucosal infection. It is uncommon in developed countries but needs recognition, so a sexual history should be taken. Other specific infections such as TB may cause septic arthritis and careful assessment of risk factors and exposure is important.

Crystal arthropathy – gout and pseudogout

Deposition of crystals in articular tissue causes inflammatory arthritis (see Figure 9.1). Gout results from the deposition of monosodium urate (MSU) crystals and pseudogout from calcium

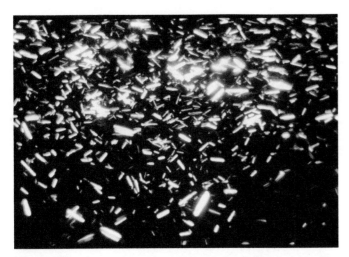

Figure 9.1 Gout crystals. By kind permission of Dr Rod Amos.

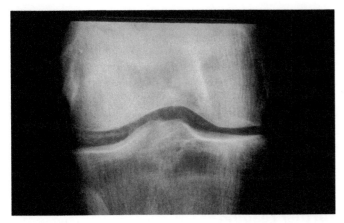

Figure 9.2 X-ray showing chondrocalcinosis of the knee. By kind permission of Dr John Winfield.

pyrophosphate dihydrate (CPPD) crystals (see Figure 9.2). Both are more common in previously damaged (e.g. osteoarthritic) joints .

Gout is the commonest form of inflammatory arthritis in men over 40. Hyperuricaemia (usually caused by renal under-excretion) is the main risk factor, although most people with hyperuricaemia will not develop gout and acute gout can occur with normal serum urate levels. Other risk factors include hypertension, family history, centripetal obesity, alcohol excess, purine excess (dietary or secondary to increased purine turnover, e.g. myeloproliferative disease) and chronic kidney disease.

Classical gout presents in the early hours of the morning with a monoarthritis affecting the lower limb – 70% are affected in the first metatarsophalangeal joint but knee, ankle and instep are commonly affected. Useful additional clues include typical history, joint erythema and hyperuricaemia. Classical gouty tophi are a feature of chronic hyperuricaemia, but provide a useful clue if discovered. The pain of gout is often excruciating, and in acute attacks, patients are usually unable to bear the slightest touch.

CPPD arthritis presents acutely as monoarticular or polyarticular pain and swelling, commonly involving knees, wrists and metacarpophalangeal joints (especially 2nd and 3rd). Distinguishing this from septic arthritis or gout can be difficult.

Trauma/haemarthrosis

In patients with increased tendency to bleed, such as those on warfarin or with haemophilia, even minor trauma can cause haemarthrosis. Blood in the articular space is very irritant and will cause intense pain such that the joint is often held immobile. A history of injury should be taken.

Reactive arthritis

Reactive arthritis (ReA) develops in genetically predisposed people exposed to a triggering infection although the precise pathogenesis is not understood. Most commonly the infective agent has affected the digestive tract (e.g. *Campylobacter*) or the urogenital tract (e.g. *Chlamydia trachomatis*) but there are multiple other possible organisms and sites of infection. A history of recent illness or infection may therefore point to this diagnosis.

ReA most commonly affects healthy young adults and there is a period of incubation of up to a month after initial infection. The arthritis which develops is sterile, peripheral, asymmetric and oligoarticular and lies on a spectrum from mild to very disabling. It is frequently associated with extra-articular features such as acute iritis, enthesitis such as achilles tendonitis and urethritis or cervicitis. Good history taking, including a detailed sexual history, is therefore the cornerstone in recognising ReA.

First presentation of a subsequent polyarthritis

Any inflammatory arthritis (for example rheumatoid arthritis or spondyloarthropathy) or connective tissue disease such as systemic lupus erythematosus may initially present with a single swollen joint and is beyond the scope of this chapter.

Other causes of an acutely swollen joint not suggested by the history

There are uncommon causes of an acutely swollen joint which should be clarified by history and examination and include tumours, rare inflammatory monoarthritis such as pigmented villo-nodular synovitis and infections such as Lyme disease, brucellosis and acute HIV infection. In the former causes, the history will usually be more protracted, and in the latter travel, social or occupational clues will help.

Case history revisited

The acute onset of swelling and pain in a large joint makes septic arthritis or crystal arthropathy most likely. His high alcohol intake points towards gout but septic arthritis must remain an important diagnosis of exclusion. The absence of trauma makes haemarthrosis very unlikely. Although there is a history of travel to Thailand, reactive arthritis is unlikely in this case because of the absence of other systemic symptoms. A first presentation of a subsequent polyarthritis cannot be discounted altogether from the history.

Examination

Apart from obvious pain in his knee, this man looks well. His temperature is 36.8°C, pulse 80 beats/minute, and blood pressure 148/94 mmHg. He cannot bear touch to his affected knee, which is

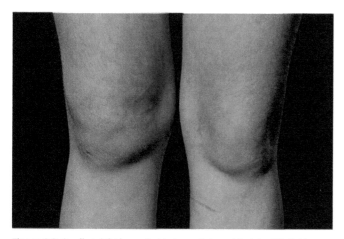

Figure 9.3 Swollen right knee. By kind permission of Dr John Winfield.

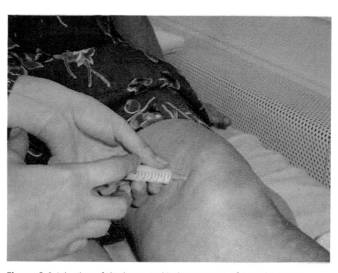

Figure 9.4 Injection of the knee. By kind permission of Dr Kelsey Jordan.

red and swollen with a moderate effusion (see Figure 9.3). The rest of his joints and physical examination are normal.

Question: Given the history and examination findings what is your principal working diagnosis?

Principal working diagnosis – gout

Management

Although gout is now the most likely diagnosis, septic arthritis should still be considered. The diagnosis of septic arthritis hinges on urgent aspiration of infected synovial fluid with prompt culture and close liaison with microbiology colleagues (see Figure 9.4). Aspiration should be an aseptic, 'no touch' technique. Bacterial yield is improved if synovial fluid is collected into blood culture bottles. Blood cultures should also be taken and estimation of C-reactive protein (CRP) is useful in monitoring subsequent response to treatment.

Microscopic examination of aspirated joint fluid also conveniently provides an opportunity to look for crystals. This analysis needs to be prompt as CPPD crystals become disrupted if left in sample jars for even a few hours.

X-rays may be very helpful where the appearance of linear or stippled calcification in articular cartilage or menisci (chondrocalcinosis) is highly suggestive of CPPD arthritis. In many cases of acute arthritis, however, the X-rays are normal.

Supporting investigations may include full blood count, biochemical parameters (including uric acid), viral screens and genitourinary screening depending on the clinical context.

Outcome

This man had a mildly raised white cell count and CRP. His knee was aspirated to dryness which produced considerable pain relief. The fluid was yellow and turbid and was sent for urgent microscopy and Gram staining. There were a large number of neutrophils but no organisms. Urate crystals were demonstrated in the synovial fluid aspirate and there was no subsequent growth on microbiological culture. He was given a diagnosis of gout and improved dramatically with non-steroidal anti-inflammatory drugs. He adjusted his alcohol intake accordingly.

Further reading

Bardin T. Gonococcal arthritis. *Best Practice and Research Clinical Rheumatology* 2003; **17**:201–208.

Coakley G, Mathews C, Field M, Jones A *et al.* BSR & BHPR, BOA, RCGP and BSAC guidelines for management of the hot swollen joint in adults. *Rheumatology* 2006; **45**:1039–1041.

Doherty M, Dacre J, Dieppe P, Snaith M. The 'GALS' locomotor system. *Annals of Rheumatic Disease* 1992; **51**:1165–1169.

Khan MA. Update on spondyloarthropathies. *Annals of Internal Medicine* 2002; **136**:896–907.

Kherani R, Shojania K. Septic arthritis in patients with pre-existing inflammatory arthritis. *Canadian Medical Journal* 2007; **176**:1605–1608.

Underwood M. Diagnosis and management of gout. *British Medical Journal* 2006; **332**:1315–1319.

CHAPTER 10

Chest Pain – Pleuritic

Claire Gardner and Kevin Jones

Question: What differential diagnosis would you consider from the history?

Pleurisy is caused by irritation of the parietal pleura as an injured or infected lung rubs against it. There are many causes of pleuritic chest pain (see Table 10.1). It is important to take a careful history to determine the speed of onset of the pain and the presence of accompanying symptoms such as cough, sputum, haemoptysis, fever, myalgia, and especially breathlessness. Pleuritic pain can change a patient's breathing pattern but it is imperative to try and establish if the patient truly feels breathless and if the breathlessness came on at the same time as the pain. It is also important to determine if the pain is made worse by movement or position and if it is accompanied by tenderness.

ABC of Emergency Differential Diagnosis. Edited by F. Morris and A. Fletcher.
© 2009 Blackwell Publishing, ISBN: 978-1-4051-7063-5.

Pneumonia

Pneumonia is one of the commonest causes of pleuritic chest pain. The definition of pneumonia includes symptoms and signs of a respiratory infection and new chest radiographic shadowing consistent with consolidation (see Figure 10.1). Supportive features in the history are cough, yellow, green or brown sputum, fever, malaise,

Table 10.1 Causes of pleuritic chest pain.

Common	Uncommon
Pneumonia	Autoimmune diseases
Pulmonary embolism	Myocardial infarction
Pneumothorax	Aortic dissection
Musculoskeletal chest pain	Oesophageal rupture
Pericarditis	Pancreatitis

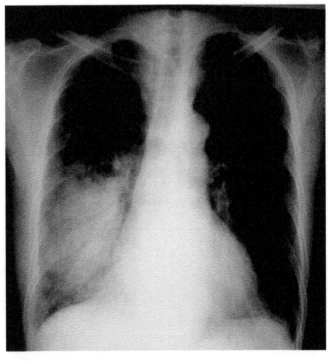

Figure 10.1 X-ray showing right lower lobe pneumonia.

headache, and a past medical history of conditions predisposing to lower respiratory tract infections, such as COPD, immuno-compromise, or alcoholism. It is important to ask about travel (for *Legionella* and rarer tropical causes) and any contacts. Breathlessness is usually a feature, but may be less obvious when fit adults with lots of respiratory reserve have a small area of infected lung.

Focal examination signs that support a diagnosis of pneumonia include dull percussion note, bronchial breathing, increased vocal resonance, crackles and pleural rub at the area of consolidation.

The commonest organism responsible for pneumonia in the UK is *Streptococcus pneumoniae* (in about 60%). This classically causes rusty brown sputum, often flecked with blood. Other cases are made up of *Haemophilus influenzae, Staphylococcus aureus, Mycoplasma pneumoniae, Legionella pneumophila,* and rarer organisms.

Pulmonary embolism (PE)

Pleuritic chest pain with PE is due to pulmonary infarction. This is usually caused by an acute small or medium embolism. Patients classically present with pleuritic chest pain, breathlessness and haemoptysis. Massive PE may present differently with syncope, central chest pain and severe dyspnoea.

PE should be considered as a possible diagnosis in almost all patients with pleuritic chest pain and is considered one of the most underdiagnosed conditions in acute medicine. Risk factors for PE are listed in Box 10.1. These are usually combined in a pre-test probability score (Wells) to guide further investigation (see Table 10.2).

Box 10.1 **Risk factors for pulmonary embolism**

- Recent surgery
- Immobility
- Previous DVT/PE
- Malignancy
- Pregnancy/puerperium
- Combined oral contraceptive pill/HRT
- Nephrotic syndrome
- Thrombophilia
- Smoking
- Long flight/car journey
- Obesity

Table 10.2 Wells score.

Clinical characteristic	Score
Clinical signs/symptoms DVT	3.0
Heart rate >100	1.5
Immobilization	1.5
Previous DVT/PE	1.5
Haemoptysis	1.0
Malignancy	1.0
PE more likely than alternative	3.0

Low probability (score ≤ 4). High probability (score >4).

The symptoms, signs and investigation results in pulmonary infarction can be very similar to pneumonia. Pulmonary infarction can cause peripheral consolidation with bronchial breathing and crackles on auscultation.

Important signs indicating possible PE include: tachypnoea, tachycardia, DVT, atrial fibrillation, and pleural rub. Signs of right ventricular strain in keeping with a diagnosis of PE include a raised JVP, right ventricular heave or loud second pulmonary heart sound (P2). The latter are usually seen in massive or sub-massive PE rather than small or moderate PE.

Musculoskeletal chest pain

Musculoskeletal chest pain is a possibility if there is a history of injury and if the pain appears to be related to movement. This is more difficult to establish than it sounds because movement of the thoracic cage can reproduce pain caused by an inflamed or infected lung. Patients can feel short of breath with musculoskeletal chest pain due to splinting of the chest and anxiety. A history of injury is not always clear, and questions about recent lifting, twisting, and sport are important.

Exacerbation of asthma or COPD

Patients with airways disease can develop exacerbations after bacterial or viral lower respiratory tract infections. They will have cough, increased expectoration of sputum, breathlessness and wheeze. The chest radiograph may be normal. Pleuritic pain may be due to co-existent pleurisy or due to musculoskeletal pain from the increased respiration and coughing which accompanies the exacerbation.

Viral pleurisy

This is a common cause of pleuritic pain. It is often in the context of a viral type illness with upper respiratory tract symptoms, myalgia and fever. There may be either a dry or productive cough. Auscultation may reveal a pleural rub (which can sometimes be felt as well as heard). The chest radiograph is usually normal although occasionally there is a small pleural effusion.

Pericarditis

In pericarditis the pain is typically pleuritic but usually retrosternal and positional. It is worse when lying down and relieved by leaning forward. There may be characteristic ECG changes (see Figure 10.2). The chest radiograph will be normal unless a pericardial effusion causes enlargement of the cardiac silhouette.

Pneumothorax

Spontaneous pneumothorax classically causes sudden onset of pleuritic chest pain and breathlessness in a previously healthy patient. The commonest findings are reduced expansion and air-entry on the side of the pneumothorax. The chest radiograph is diagnostic (see Figure 10.3). It usually arises in young, slim males, or in those with COPD, and is sometimes linked to an inherited condition such as Ehlers–Danlos syndrome.

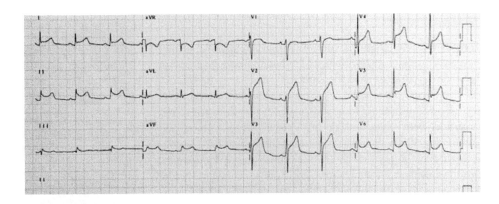

Figure 10.2 ECG in pericarditis.

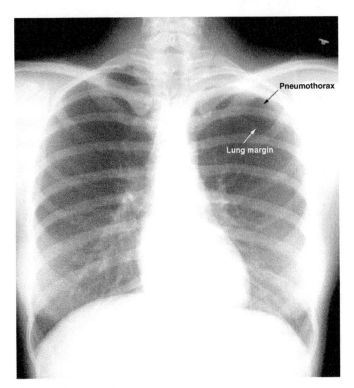

Figure 10.3 Pneumothorax.

Case history revisited

On revisiting the case history the diagnosis is not immediately obvious, and all of the conditions discussed are possible. The most serious diagnosis to consider is pulmonary embolism. The fact that the pain arose outside an immediate context of infective symptoms and is associated with breathlessness means that pulmonary embolism still needs to be definitely excluded. There is also exposure to possible hospital acquired infections.

This patient has a significant PE risk factor having had a total hip replacement 2 weeks ago. The swollen leg may represent a deep vein thrombosis (DVT) although after a total hip replacement the affected leg will usually be swollen anyway. Her Wells score is 8.5 putting her in the high probability group. She has symptoms and signs of a possible DVT (3), haemoptysis (1), immobilization (1.5) and PE is more likely than the alternative diagnosis (3).

Musculoskeletal chest pain is a possibility here due to the history of injury and in that the pain appears related to movement. This should be kept as reserve differential diagnosis because PE and pneumonia are more likely.

Examination

She has a good colour, temperature is 37.8°C, pulse 90 beats/minute, blood pressure 130/75 mmHg, respiratory rate 20 breaths/minute, and oxygen saturations 92% on air.

Pulse is regular, of normal volume and her jugular venous pressure (JVP) is visible 2 cm above the suprasternal notch. The apex beat is not displaced and there is no right ventricular heave. Heart sounds are normal with no murmurs heard.

Chest examination reveals equal expansion, resonant percussion note throughout and on auscultation there is a mild wheeze bilaterally. There is some chest wall tenderness but the pain is not clearly reproducible. Her abdomen is soft and non-tender. There is bilateral ankle oedema. The left leg is diffusely swollen but not red or tender.

Question: Given the history and examination findings what is your principal working diagnosis?

Principal working diagnosis – PE

This patient is tachypnoeic and hypoxic. There are no signs of consolidation and there are pointers toward possible DVT. Pneumonia and musculoskeletal chest pain are both possible but less likely: the fever keeps pneumonia as an important differential but this may also be seen in PE. The wheeze is probably due to COPD; this may be exacerbated by infection. Wheeze can also sometimes be heard in PE.

There is some chest wall tenderness and musculoskeletal chest pain remains a possibility but this patient has low oxygen saturations and an increased respiratory rate indicating lung pathology. Musculoskeletal pain is a diagnosis of exclusion in this case. In patients with suspected PE, chest pain reproduced by palpation is not associated with a lower prevalence of PE and we should not be misguided by chest wall tenderness in this case.

Patients with COPD may be chronically hypoxic and for some, saturations of 92% on air are normal. However, this patient is normally independent, she only has mild COPD and she is breathless. These saturations are very unlikely to be normal in her case.

Management

Oxygen must be given via controlled delivery to maintain her oxygen saturations ≥92%. Nebulised salbutamol and ipratropium bromide should be given as she is wheezy.

Intravenous access should be obtained and blood tests requested: full blood count should look particularly at the white cell count, urea and electrolytes, and clotting screen. Blood cultures and sputum for culture should be collected as this patient has a fever.

Arterial blood gases should be performed to look for hypoxia, ideally while she is breathing room air if she is well enough. D-dimer is not required as she has a high probability Wells score, but for low probability this is a useful screening tool. An ECG may show signs of pulmonary embolus (see Box 10.2, Figure 10.4).

She needs a chest X-ray to look for consolidation indicating pneumonia. There may be signs of PE on the chest X-ray, such as a small effusion, focal infiltrates, segmental collapse or raised hemidiaphragm but the most common finding is for it to be normal.

Investigation of PE begins with a Doppler ultrasound scan of the deep veins of her swollen leg. If she has a DVT it can be assumed, based on her symptoms, that she has a PE. If there is no DVT then

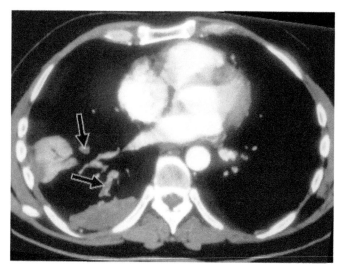

Figure 10.5 CTPA showing pulmonary embolus (arrows).

a computerised tomographic pulmonary angiogram (CTPA) should be performed regardless of whether the chest X-ray shows consolidation (see Figure 10.5). Her Wells score is high and it is possible she has both PE and pneumonia.

Outcome

This patient had a raised white cell count. Arterial blood gases showed hypoxia with a normal pH and slightly low carbon dioxide. Her ECG showed a sinus tachycardia and chest X-ray was clear. Leg Doppler confirmed a DVT so CTPA was not needed. The final diagnosis was PE secondary to recent orthopaedic surgery. She was anticoagulated with low molecular weight heparin and subsequently with warfarin.

Further reading

Boon NA, Colledge NR, Walker BR, Hunter JAA. *Davidson's Principles and Practice of Medicine*, 20th edition. Churchill Livingstone, Edinburgh, 2006.

British Thoracic Society guidelines for the management of suspected acute pulmonary embolism. *Thorax* 2003; **58**: 470–483.

Kasper DL, Braunwald E, Hauser S. *Harrison's Principles of Internal Medicine*, 16th edition. McGraw-Hill Medical Publishing, New York, 2005.

Warrell DA, Cox TM, Firth JD, Benz EJ Jr (Eds). *Oxford Textbook of Medicine*, Fourth Edition. Oxford University Press, Oxford, 2003.

West S, Chapman S, Robinson G, Stradling J. *Oxford Handbook of Respiratory Medicine*, Fourth Edition. Oxford University Press, Oxford, 2003.

Box 10.2 **Possible ECG signs of pulmonary embolus**

- Sinus tachycardia (most commonly)
- Atrial fibrillation
- Right bundle branch block
- Right axis deviation
- SI,QIII,TIII (S wave lead I, Q wave and inverted T in lead III)
- T inversion in V1–V4

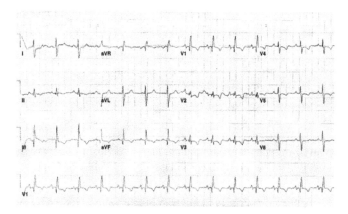

Figure 10.4 ECG showing right heart strain.

CHAPTER 11

Dizziness

Scott Davison

Question: What differential diagnosis would you consider from the history?

When assessing a patient with dizziness clarification of the points in Box 11.1 are important.

The first issue is to discriminate between different types of dizziness, which are broadly, vertiginous and non-vertiginous. Patients with vertigo, a specific complaint, often find it difficult to clearly articulate their symptoms. Vertigo is a false perception of movement. The sensation of vertigo results from unilateral damage anywhere in the vestibular system. Table 11.1 provides examples of how patients describes their dizziness. The questions in Box 11.2 may help patients describe the sensation experienced. The duration of the vertigo is the single most important factor in elucidating the cause of the vertigo (see Box 11.3).

Box 11.1 Important points to clarify when assessing a patient with dizziness

- A clear description of the dizziness
- Its duration
- Accompanying symptoms
- Provoking factors
- Previous episodes

Table 11.1 Examples of how patients describe their dizziness.

Vertiginous	Non-vertiginous
Spinning	Light-headed
Everything moving	Floaty
Tumbling	Passing out
As if really drunk	Vision went grey
As if got off fairground ride	Woozy
Seasick	Spaced-out
Rocking	Empty-headed
Things are at an angle	

Box 11.2 Questions that may help the patient describe the sensation experienced

1 Is it like you are about to fall over, or pass out?
2 Does it feel as if you have been spinning around, or as if you have stood up too quickly?
3 Do you feel you may loose awareness of your surroundings, or do they appear to be moving?

Box 11.3 The duration of nystagmus is the single most important factor in elucidating the cause of the vertigo

- Seconds – benign paroxysmal positional vertigo
- Minutes to an hour – migraine/TIA
- Several hours – Ménière's disease/TIA
- Several days – Vestibular neuritis/CVA/demyelination

As there is some overlap, further questions will be required to help discriminate between the differing causes. Obviously, in the acute presentation of recent onset, one cannot predict how long the vertigo will last.

A focused history will elucidate any important associated symptoms which may help to refine the diagnosis. For instance, associated deafness and tinnitus suggest an otological cause, whereas diplopia dysarthria and dysphagia point strongly to a neurological disease. Table 11.2 gives some categories of dizziness and the likelihood of certain associated presenting symptoms. A vertiginous patient will always want to keep their head still either sat up with chin tilted forward, so as to limit stimulation of the lateral semicircular canals, or lying on the side of the unaffected ear.

ABC of Emergency Differential Diagnosis. Edited by F. Morris and A. Fletcher. © 2009 Blackwell Publishing, ISBN: 978-1-4051-7063-5.

Table 11.2 Some categories of dizziness and the likelihood of certain associated presenting symptoms.

Symptom	Cardiovascular	Otological	Neurological	Anxiety	Presyncope
Nausea	+	+++	+	+/–	+
Vomiting	+	++	+	+/–	+/–
Breathlessness	++	–	–	++	–
Palpitations	++	–	+/–	++	+/–
Chest pain or tightness	++	–	–	+	–
Tinnitus	+/–	++	+	+	+
Acute deafness or pressure in ears	–	++ (unilateral)	+ (bilateral)	–	–
Dysarthria	–	–	+++	–	–
Greying or loss of vision	+	–	+	–	++
Diplopia	–	–	++	–	–
Ataxia	–	+	+++	–	–
Pallor	++	+/–	–	–	++
Paraesthesia	–	–	++	+	+/–

Key: +++ Almost universal. ++ Very common. + Common. +/– May be present. – Unlikely.

It is always worth asking whether the patient has had vertigo before, and if so, to describe previous episodes. Multiple episodes point towards a diagnosis of Ménière's disease, migraine, transient ischaemic attack (TIA) or benign paroxysmal positional vertigo (BPPV), rather than acute labyrinthitis, or vestibular neuronitis.

Taking the above into account, and the information provided in this patient's history, the differential diagnosis should include the conditions below.

Acute unilateral peripheral vestibulopathy (a.k.a. vestibular neuronitis)

The cause of this is unknown, but it remains the commonest cause of the first episode of prolonged vertigo. Many different terms are used to describe the syndrome of acute, apparently idiopathic, unilateral vestibular failure but given that the pathology is unconfirmed, acute peripheral vestibulopathy (APV) would seem the best term. The onset is spontaneous, associated with nausea and vomiting, persisting for more than 24 hours, with ataxic gait, horizontal nystagmus, with the fast phase towards the *unaffected* ear, and the absence of hearing loss or tinnitus. Ear examination and the Rinne's and Weber's tuning fork tests are typically normal (see Box 11.4 and Figure 11.1).

By definition, APV must last over 24 hours, so at this stage of assessment, it remains in the differential.

Ménière's disease

This is due to episodic increase in pressure of the endolymphatic fluid in the labyrinth and cochlea. The classical presentation is with a prodrome of unilateral aural pressure/fullness, with subsequent onset of vertigo, which lasts several hours and there is associated unilateral deafness and tinnitus, lasting days and sometimes weeks. Note that patients may only perceive their hearing loss as a 'blocked feeling' in the ear. Furthermore, as it is usually low frequency loss, it may not be noted at all. Initially there may be episodes of solitary vertigo, before the recurrent pattern of vertigo and hearing loss becomes evident over time.

In the typical presentation, one would anticipate a bilateral Rinne's positive (i.e. normal) and Weber's lateralising towards the unaffected side (abnormal).

In this case, the absence of prior episodes and accompanying otological symptoms (aural fullness/pressure, hearing loss and tinnitus) would be atypical for Ménière's disease, though this attack could be the first episode.

Focal migraine

This condition is under-diagnosed and is typified by the complaint of recurrent unprovoked (i.e. not triggered by positional change) vertigo lasting up to around an hour, without hearing loss or tinnitus. A history or family history of any form of migraine, especially focal, would favour this diagnosis. There may be triggers such as menstruation (a drop in oestrogen), altered sleep pattern, life event 'stress' or similar, that triggered the attack.

As the patient has migraine the diagnosis should be considered, though the duration of the attack would be atypical.

Cerebellar TIA/stroke

This man has a number of risk factors for cerebral vascular disease and a vascular cause for his symptoms should be considered. A careful history and examination is required to identify any neurological deficit.

In the absence of associated neurological symptoms or signs such as dysarthria, diplopia or ataxia, a vertebrobasilar vascular cause is rather unlikely. Note, however that, if there is a short history of transient bilateral hearing loss with each episode lasting minutes,

Box 11.4 **Rinne's and Weber's tuning fork tests**

Modified Rinne's test (512 Hz tuning fork required – with baseplate and ideally a quiet space)
1 Explain that you are going to place the fork in two positions and you want the patient to tell you which is the loudest.
2 Lightly activate the fork, and place on the mastoid area for around 3 seconds, with the vibrating axis of the fork vertical.
3 Next place the fork around 15 cm from the ear for a similar period, with the vibrating axis in line with the external auditory meatus.
4 Do the same on the other ear.

Results and interpretation
1 Louder alongside ear/both ears: air conduction (AC), louder than bone condition (BC). This is known as Rinne's positive and is normal. This excludes a significant conductive loss.
2 Louder on the mastoid: BC is louder than AC. This could be either:
  • A true Rinne's negative due to a conductive hearing loss in the ipsilateral ear or
  • False Rinne's negative, when the ipsilateral ear has a severe sensorineural deafness, but the patient responds to the sound transmitting through the skull to the contralateral cochlea.
In order to discriminate, one can either repeat the Rinne's test whilst 'masking' the contralateral ear – essentially 'distracting' that ear by making circular rubbing movements over the tragus, see below

Weber's test (512 Hz tuning fork required – with base plate, and ideally a quiet space)
1 Explain that you are going to place the tuning fork on their head and you want to know if the sound appears louder in one ear than the other.
2 Moderately strongly activate the fork and place for 5 seconds on the vertex, vibrating the axis in line with the ears.

Results and interpretation
1 Sound is central or patient equivocal: Weber's normal.
Sound heard louder in one ear. Either the patient has a conductive loss in the side to which the sound localised, or they have a sensorineal loss in the contralateral side. The Rinne's test carried out beforehand should have already given you an idea, and allow you to discern between these possibilities.

then this could be due to TIAs in this territory. Otological causes of vertigo are invariably associated with horizontal nystagmus whereas the absence of nystagmus or unusual forms of nystagmus, e.g. vertical, point to a potential vascular cause.

Other causes of dizziness not suggested by the history
Benign paroxysmal positional vertigo
This common condition describes brief vertigo of no longer than 1 minute and usually less than 20 seconds, provoked by change in posture. Whilst the majority of such cases are idiopathic, some follow head injury or labyrinthitis.

Perilymph fistula
This is thought to occur when the *round* window (not the tympanic membrane) perforates. It usually is provoked when someone has been straining, or diving, and also results in hearing loss. It may

also occur in the setting of chronic suppurative middle ear disease. None of these symptoms are present in our man's history.

Labyrinthitis
This term should be reserved for where there is evidence of acute otitis media and hearing loss accompanying the vertigo. Such patients require admission to the ENT department.

Vestibular schwannoma /posterior fossa tumour
These conditions rarely present with isolated vertigo. The typical presenting features are progressive unilateral hearing loss and/or tinnitus. The slow growth of these tumours allows a process of central compensation to occur, which can manifest as a sensation of vague imbalance, but not vertigo. Note, however, that very rarely these tumours may present with acute hearing loss.

Case history revisited

Further questioning is required to help this man clearly articulate the spinning sensation so there is no doubt that he is complaining of vertigo. Ask about fullness in the ear as well as deafness, and confirm there are no focal neurological symptoms such as dysarthria, diplopia, etc. The examination should specifically look for nystagmus, ear pathology and focal neurology. Deafness and vestibular function can be clinically assessed using the Weber's, Rinne's, Romberg's and head-thrust tests (see Boxes 11.3–11.5; Figures 11.2–11.4).

Examination

This man is sat still with his eyes closed. He is sweaty, with vomit on his clothing. Observations show pulse 84/minute, regular, blood pressure 146/82 mmHg.

He has no spontaneous nystagmus*, but there is subtle right-beating nystagmus on lateral gaze to the right. He is (reluctantly) able to stand, with his eyes open and feet together. He falls to the left on Romberg testing and is unable to complete the Unterberger test (see Box 11.6 for explanation). The tympanic membranes are normal.

His speech is normal, there is no complaint of double vision on assessing the cranial nerves or evidence of loss of co-ordination. The remainder of the neurological examination is normal.

His tuning fork tests show Rinne's positive bilaterally and Weber's central (i.e. they are normal). The head-thrust test is positive to the left. This confirms the diagnosis of peripheral left-sided vestibular failure and is against a 'central' cause such as stroke. This is because the oculo-vestibular reflex remains intact in the latter, but is obviously disrupted in acute peripheral vestibular failure (see Table 11.3).

Question: Given the history and examination findings what is your principal working diagnosis?

Principal working diagnosis – acute peripheral vestibulopathy
Despite his risk factors for cerebral vascular disease, the absence of any neurological symptoms or signs with the exception of nystagmus all point to an otological cause for his symptoms.

Air conduction (AC) is louder than bone conduction (BC) Weber's central

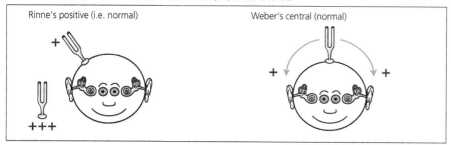

BC is louder than AC. This is either (a) true Rinne's negative or (b) false Rinne's negative

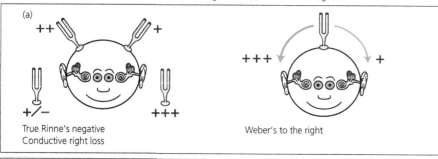

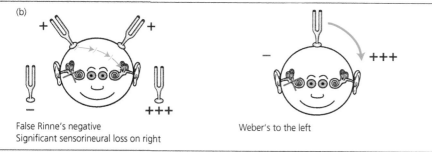

An alternative way to discriminate between true and false Rinne's negative is to mask the contralateral ear, e.g. by occluding the external meatus by rubbing the tragus (tragal rub) in rapid circular movements (c)

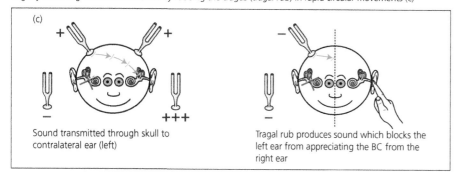

Figure 11.1 Rinne's and Weber's tuning fork tests: results and interpretation.

Table 11.3 Underlying causes of dizziness.

Pathology	Clinical test		
	Head thrust	**Able to stand unaided, eyes open?**	**Nystagmus**
Unilateral APV	Positive (towards side of lesion)	Yes	Fixed, unidirectional, horizontal, suppressed by optic fixation
Cerebellar ischaemia	Negative	No	Often vertical, or multi-directional, spontaneous, not readily suppressed

Box 11.5 **The head-thrust test and the head impulse test**

Head-thrust test (Figure 11.2)

Normal head-thrust test to the left (a and b)
Starting position (a) places subject's head 30 degrees into cervical flexion; eyes are focused on the target (examiner's forehead). Head is thrust *rapidly*, 10–20 degrees to the left (b). Upon stopping the head thrust, the eyes are still on target and *no* corrective saccade (bringing eyes back to target) is observed.

Abnormal head trust test to the right (c–e)
Starting position as before (c). Head is thrust *rapidly* to the right, the eyes lose their target and move with the head (d). The subject must make a corrective saccade (small arrows) to bring the eyes back to target (e). In this case, the right vestibular-ocular reflex is abnormal. Repeat three times to each side, randomly; a majority (i.e. two or more) abnormal response is taken as pathological.

The head impulse test (Figure 11.3)

The examiner turns the patient's head as rapidly as possible about 15 degrees to one side and observes the ability of the patient to keep fixating on a distant target. The patient illustrated has a right peripheral vestibular lesion with a severe loss of right lateral semicircular canal function. While the examiner turns the patient's head toward the normal left side (top row) the patient is able to keep fixating on target. By contrast, when the examiner turns the patient's head to the right the vestibulo-ocular reflex fails and the patient cannot keep fixating on target (e) so that she needs to make a voluntary rapid eye movement – that is, a saccade, back to target (f) after the head impulse has finished; this can be easily observed by the examiner. It is essential that the head is turned as rapidly as possible as otherwise smooth pursuit eye movements will compensate for the head turn.

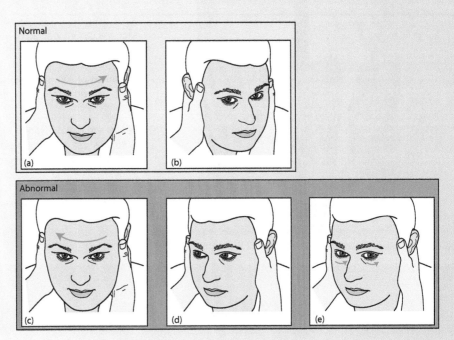

Figure 11.2 The head-thrust test.

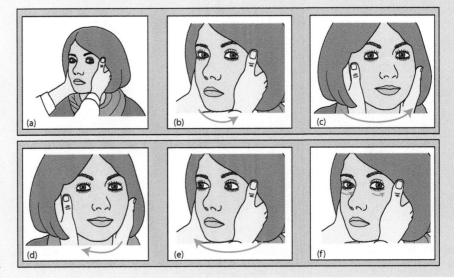

Figure 11.3 The head-impulse test.

Box 11.6 **The Romberg test and the Unterberger test**

Romberg test (Figure 11.4)

This test is classically one of joint position sense, but can also test the vestibular system (vestibulo-spinal reflex). Stand close to the subject so that in the event of a fall you are able to catch them. Reassure them that you are there. An assistant may be required for large patients. The patient stands feet together, arms by sides with eyes open. If they cannot complete this test, they cannot proceed to the Romberg. Next, ask them to close their eyes.

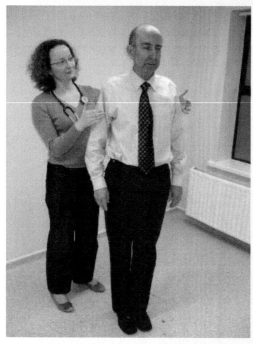

Figure 11.4 The Romberg test.

Results and interpretation

1 Cannot stand feet together with eyes open (unable to undertake Romberg): this usually indicates severe loss of cerebellar function.
2 Stands with eyes open and closed: 'Romberg negative' – normal.
3 Stands with eyes open, sways significantly (or falls) with eyes closed: 'Romberg positive' – this indicates that the patient is relying heavily on their visual input in order to maintain balance. The following are possibilities: (a) Problem with proprioceptive information reaching the cerebellum either through peripheral neuropathy in the lower limbs, or dorsal column lesions. (b) Vestibular lesion, in which case the patient tends to fall consistently towards the pathological side. These two can be discriminated by testing sensory modalities in the lower limbs.
4 Stands with eyes open, sways fore and aft with eyes closed: this is typical of mild (chronic) cerebellar pathology.

Unterberger test ('stepping test') (Figure 11.5)

The patient is asked to 'walk' on the spot, for 50 steps or 30 seconds, with eyes closed, hands clasped and arms extended. Ensure there is adequate room and be ready to catch the patient. It is useful to align the patient with an object to help you discern the degree of movement. Avoid pointing the patient at bright light sources, as these may guide the patient. If the patient has locomotor problems/ asymmetry of gait, these preclude testing. It is useful to think of the hands of a clock face, with '5-past' equating to 30 degrees, '10-past', 60 degrees, etc.

Results and interpretation

1 Rotates <30 degrees: normal (Figure 11.5b).
2 Rotates 30–45 degrees: borderline. Suggest rotate the patient 180 degrees and repeat, looking for consistency. Vestibular lesion on the ipsilateral side.
3 Rotates >45 degrees: abnormal. Turns to the pathological side (Figure 11.5c).

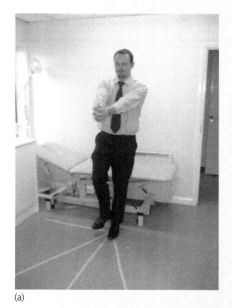

(a)

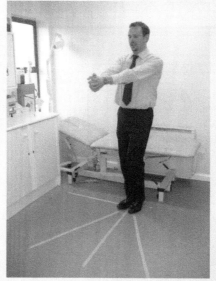

(b)

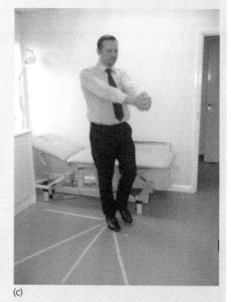

(c)

Figure 11.5 The Unterberger test. (a) Starting position. (b) Normal (turning <30 degrees after 50 steps). (c) Abnormal (turns >45 degrees to the left) (suggests relative hypofunction of the left vestibular system, e.g. in acute peripheral vestibulopathy).

Management

A vestibular sedative should be administered, preferably by mouth, but a parenteral route will often be required, e.g. prochlorperazine 12.5 mg i.m. An alternative for those with a history of previous dystonic reactions, or other contraindications, would be diazepam, which may be administered rectally, when the oral route is not possible (10–20 mg 12-hourly) when necessary. It may be given slowly i.v. (5–10 mg, at 5 mg/minute) but be aware of the potential for respiratory depression, and close supervision and pulse oximetry should be used.

Patients who do not respond to treatment or those who live alone may require hospital admission. Those managed at home should be issued with a small supply of vestibular sedatives, such as prochlorperazine 5 mg three times a day. It is very important that patients do not use vestibular sedatives for a protracted period, as this appears to hinder the central compensating mechanisms that allow them recovery. They should be advised to stop, or weaned off them after 1 week. Follow up should be arranged through the local ENT/Audiovestibular Medicine Clinic.

Most patients make a full symptomatic recovery from unilateral APV, even though asymmetry of vestibular function may be evident on clinical testing. In those other cases, a sense of disequilibrium (intolerance of movement causing momentary imbalance) may arise and loss of confidence occur where the visual cues are reduced, such as in the dark, or when making rapid movements, e.g. turning the head before crossing the road. In such cases, vestibular rehabilitation exercises should be deployed.

Outcome

This man responded to treatment with prochlorperazine and was managed at home. Given his occupation was HGV driving he was advised not to go back to work for at the very least a week, and to seek the advice of his GP as to whether he is fit to return thereafter.

Note

*Note that nystagmus of otological origin is easily suppressed by optic fixation. Thus it may only be detected if this is removed by using specialised Frenzel glasses which have 'jamjar-bottom' type lenses through which it is impossible to focus. Alternatively moving the patient to a darkened room, or covering one eye, whilst undertaking fundoscopy on the other, will also unmask it.

Further reading

Axford J, O'Callaghan C. *Medicine*, Second Edition. Blackwell Publishing, Oxford, 2004.

Knot A, Polmear A. *Practical General Practice: Guidelines for Effective Clinical Management*, Fourth Edition. Butterworth-Heinemann, Oxford, 2004.

Ramrakha P, Moore K. *Oxford Handbook of Acute Medicine*, Second Edition. Oxford University Press, Oxford, 2004.

Simon C, Everitt H, Kendrick T. *Oxford Handbook of General Practice*, Second Edition. Oxford University Press, Oxford, 2002.

Tintinalli J, Kelen G, Stapczynski S, *et al. Emergency Medicine: A Comprehensive Study Guide*, Sixth Edition. McGraw-Hill, New York, 2003.

Wyatt JP, Illingworth R, Graham C, *et al. Oxford Handbook of Emergency Medicine*, Third Edition. Oxford University Press, Oxford, 2006.

CHAPTER 12

The Intoxicated Patient

Sue Croft

CASE HISTORY

A 35-year-old man presents with confusion, blood around his mouth and a cut across his forehead. He thinks that he fell over and banged his head the previous evening after drinking 2 litres of vodka (i.e. 80 units of alcohol – see Table 12.1). He woke up this morning on the floor in his flat and cannot recall any other events. It is difficult to elicit whether he lost consciousness though he has vomited twice. On further questioning he tells you that he drinks approximately 2 litres of vodka every day and that he has 'numb feet' which a specialist has attributed to the alcohol. He denies any other illnesses or medication.

Table 12.1 Alcohol content of some common beverages.

Beverage type	Quantity (ml)	Alcohol content (units)
Lager/beer	568 (1 pint)	2.0
Cider (regular)	568 (1 pint)	2.8
Wine (12% ABV)	175 (1 medium glass)	2.4
Alcopops	275 (1 bottle)	1.4
Vodka, whisky, gin	25 (1 pub measure)	1.0
Port, sherry, martini	50 (1 pub measure)	1.0

Question: What differential diagnosis would you consider from the history?

There are a number of potential causes for his condition which relate either to the acute or chronic abuse of alcohol.

Hypoglycaemia

Normally plasma glucose level is maintained between 3.6 and 5.8 mmol/l. Plasma glucose levels of less than 3 mmol/l cause over-activity of the sympathetic nervous system and neuroglycopenia (hypoglycaemic effect on the brain). These produce symptoms described in the clinical scenario and often mimic alcohol withdrawal or intoxication (see Table 12.3).

Hypoglycaemia is often associated with diabetes and its treatments but is also associated with excessive alcohol intake in non-diabetics. It is thought that alcohol causes redistribution of pancreatic blood flow causing increased insulin production.

Post-ictal state

The post-ictal state is defined as the state of altered consciousness occurring immediately after a seizure. It lasts between 5 minutes and several hours and is characterised by drowsiness, confusion, nausea, hypertension, headache or migraine and other disorienting symptoms. In addition, emergence from this period is often accompanied by amnesia or other memory defects. It is during this period that the brain recovers from the 'trauma' of the seizure.

Box 12.1 **Alcohol**

The euphoric effect of alcohol from fermented berries has been recognised for thousands of years. Today, drinking alcohol is a popular social activity. Regular consumption of small amounts of alcohol provides some health benefits. There is evidence that it protects against ischaemic heart disease and may also offer some protection against ischaemic stroke, gallstones and reduce the risk of type 2 diabetes and Alzheimer's disease.

The UK government recommend that:
- *Men* should drink no more than 21 units of alcohol per week (and no more than four units in any one day).
- *Women* should drink no more than 14 units of alcohol per week (and no more than three units in any one day).

In the UK, over 9 million people drink more than the recommended amounts, at levels which put their health at risk. High levels of alcohol consumption lead to physical, psychological and social problems (see Table 12.2). Alcohol causes nearly 10% of all ill health and premature death in Europe.

Excessive alcohol ingestion lowers the seizure threshold, making those with epilepsy more likely to fit. It can also cause seizures in non-epileptic individuals, due to acute intoxication or alcohol withdrawal.

Acute alcohol withdrawal

Symptoms and signs of alcohol withdrawal usually occur in those who have abused alcohol on a daily basis for at least 3 months, or those who have consumed large quantities for at least a week.

ABC of Emergency Differential Diagnosis. Edited by F. Morris and A. Fletcher. © 2009 Blackwell Publishing, ISBN: 978-1-4051-7063-5.

Table 12.2 Medical problems related to alcohol.

System				
Gastrointestinal	*Liver* Fatty infiltration Alcoholic hepatitis Cirrhosis Liver failure Liver cancer	*Upper GI tract* Reflux oesophagitis Mallory – Weiss tear Oesophageal cancer Gastritis Peptic ulcers	*Other* Malabsorption Pancreatitis Malnutrition	
Neurological	*Acute intoxication* Blackouts Seizures	*Persistent damage* Korsakoff's syndrome Wernicke's encephalopathy Cerebellar degeneration Dementia	*Withdrawal* Tremor Hallucinations Seizures	*Other* Haemorrhage – subarachnoid, traumatic subdural Myopathy Neuropathy
Cardiovascular/ Respiratory	*Cardiovascular* Atrial fibrillation Hypertension Cardiomyopathy	*Respiratory* Aspiration pneumonia		
Other	*Psychiatric* Depression Anxiety disorders Schizophrenia	*Co-dependence* Marijuana addiction Cocaine addiction Smoking	*Trauma*	

Table 12.3 Symptoms of hypoglycaemia.

Sympathetic overactivity	Neuroglycopenia
Tachycardia Palpitations Sweating	Confusion Slurred speech Focal neurological defects (stroke-like syndrome)
Anxiety Pallor Tremor	Seizures Coma

Table 12.4 Alcohol withdrawal symptoms and signs.

Severity	Timing of last alcohol	Features
Mild	Within 24 hours	Tremulousness (shakes) Insomnia Anxiety Nausea
Moderate	24–36 hours	Sweating Tachycardia Irritability Hallucinations Seizures
Severe	>48 hours	'Delirium tremens'

They can start as soon as 8–12 hours after the most recent alcohol ingestion. The symptoms are usually relieved by drinking more alcohol and vary across a wide spectrum from mild nausea and minor tremulousness through to life-threatening seizures and delirium tremens (see Table 12.4).

Hallucinations occur in approximately 25% of patients withdrawing from alcohol. Symptoms consist of predominantly visual and tactile hallucinations. In the early stage, the patients recognise hallucinations. However, in the advanced stage, these hallucinations are perceived as real and may provoke extreme fear and anxiety. The patient can be seen pulling at imaginary objects, clothing, and sheets, for example.

Seizures occur in 23–33% of patients with significant alcohol withdrawal. They are usually brief, generalised, tonic-clonic without an aura. Most seizures terminate spontaneously or are easily controlled with a benzodiazepine.

Delirium tremens occurs in 5% of individuals withdrawing from alcohol within 24–72 hours after last ingestion. It is characterised by altered mental status – disorientation, confusion, delusions and severe agitation. There is associated fever, sweating and tachycardia. Untreated it has a mortality of 15% from arrhythmias (secondary to acidosis, electrolyte disturbance) and intercurrent illness.

Head injury causing intracranial pathology

Head injuries are often associated with excessive alcohol. In fact, alcohol use is thought to be a contributing factor in 50% of all adults with traumatic brain injuries. Excessive alcohol increases both the likelihood of injury and the seriousness of injury.

Chronic excessive alcohol use may cause decreased platelets and impaired clotting factor production by the liver. These patients are more likely to suffer from an intracranial haematoma from apparently minimal trauma and must be managed with care.

Symptoms and signs of serious head injury may occur immediately or may develop over hours after the injury. Some symptoms of head injury, such as amnesia, decreased conscious level and vomiting can be mistakenly attributed to alcohol excess and these patients must be assessed and investigated/observed as appropriate.

NICE have issued guidance as to which patients with head injury need urgent CT imaging, i.e. within 1 hour (see Box 12.2).

Acute thiamine deficiency

Chronic alcohol use, particularly when associated with malnutrition, can cause vitamin B1 (thiamine) deficiency. Thiamine deficiency causes damage to the mamillary bodies, cranial nerve nuclei, thalamus and cerebellum, termed Wernicke's encephalopathy, a triad of:

1 Encephalopathy (disorientation, agitation, indifference and inattentiveness, short term memory loss)
2 Occulomotor disturbance (nystagmus, lateral rectus palsy)
3 Ataxic gait

To diagnose Wernicke's encephalopathy, however, it is not necessary to have all three components present.

To protect against Wernicke's encephalopathy intravenous thiamine should be administered to any patient who is confused, with a history of alcohol abuse. If the blood sugar is also low, it is important to administer glucose with the thiamine treatment. If Wernicke's encephalopathy is not treated the confusion is liable to progress to stupor or death.

Korsakoff's psychosis is a late neuropsychiatric manifestation of Wernicke's encephalopathy. It is characterised by confusion, confabulation and amnesia (anterograde and retrograde). The memory problems associated with Korsakoff's syndrome are largely irreversible.

Box 12.2 NICE guidelines – indications for urgent CT head scan in head injuries.

- GCS <13 on initial assessment in the Emergency Department
- GCS <15 when assessed in the Emergency Department 2 hours post injury
- Suspected open or depressed skull fracture
- Any sign of basal skull fracture – haemotympanum, 'panda' eyes, cerebrospinal fluid leakage from ears or nose, Battle's sign (bruising to the mastoid area)
- Post-traumatic seizure
- Focal neurological defect
- >1 episode of vomiting
- Amnesia or loss of consciousness *and* coagulopathy

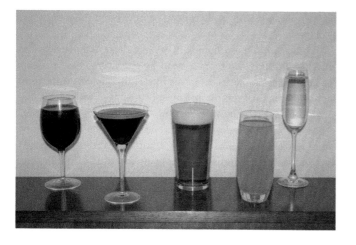

Table 12.5 Effects of acute alcohol ingestion.

Stage	Effect
Euphoria	Overall improvement in mood, becoming more self-confident and daring. Attention span shortens and judgement becomes impaired
Lethargy	Sleepiness, difficulty understanding or remembering things. Reactions slow and body movements become uncoordinated
Confusion	Profound confusion, disorientation, heightened emotional state – aggression, withdrawal or overly affectionate. Nausea and vomiting
Stupor	GCS fluctuates between 3 and 13
Coma	GCS 3/15, pupil reflexes to light diminished, pulse and respiratory rate lowers

Acute alcohol intoxication

Alcohol affects the brain like an anaesthetic. The effects of alcohol depend on the amount ingested (see Table 12.5).

Measuring the serum alcohol level has limited use – it confirms approximately how much alcohol has been ingested but does not exclude other important causes which may co-exist.

This diagnosis is not suggested by the history.

Alcoholic ketosis

This is an acute metabolic acidosis that typically occurs in people who chronically abuse alcohol and have a recent history of binge drinking, little or no food intake, and persistent vomiting.

Patients typically present with nausea, vomiting and abdominal pain. They are usually hypotensive, tachycardic and tachypnoeic with the fruity odour of ketones present on their breath. They are usually alert and lucid, but may have mild confusion.

Investigations show a raised anion gap metabolic acidosis, with normal lactate and raised serum and urine ketone levels.

Systemic infections

People with chronic alcohol dependence are relatively immuno-compromised, malnourished and more commonly exposed to infectious agents (e.g. tuberculosis) than others. Infections, in particular of the nervous system, e.g. meningitis, encephalitis, can present with non-specific confusion and vomiting.

Case history revisited

Revisiting the case, the diagnosis is not immediately obvious. This man regularly drinks excessive amounts of alcohol and presents more than 12 hours after ingesting a large amount of alcohol. This late presentation would not be typical for a presentation of acute alcohol intoxication.

On examination, his Glasgow Coma Score (GCS) is 14/15 (E4, M6, V4) – he is confused and disorientated to time and person. His observations are: blood pressure 160/100 mmHg, pulse 120 beats/minute, respiratory rate 20 breaths/minute and blood glucose (meter) 4.5 mmol. He appears sweaty and is irritable, but allows you to perform a limited examination.

He has a 4 cm cut to his forehead (partial thickness) with some surrounding swelling, but no bogginess. He has no post-auricular bruising, haemotympanum, 'panda' eyes or evidence of a cerebrospinal fluid leak.

He has slurred speech and a tremor at rest. Peripheral nervous system examination reveals normal power, tone, reflexes and sensation but coordination is impaired with dysdiadokinesia. Nystagmus is noted on eye examination, otherwise cranial nerves are intact.

Whilst you are examining him he appears to be becoming more agitated. He is pulling at the sheets and grabbing out at the air periodically and is becoming less cooperative.

Question: Given the history and examination findings what is your principal working diagnosis?

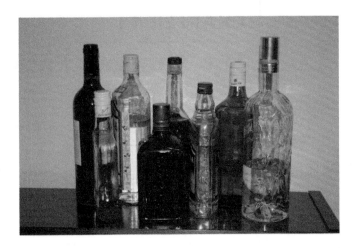

Principal working diagnosis – Acute alcohol withdrawal – though one needs to exclude intracranial pathology and acute thiamine deficiency

The most likely diagnosis for this patient is acute alcohol withdrawal. He is sweaty and tachycardic, has a tremor and is becoming increasingly agitated. Pulling at his sheets and grabbing at the air may be signs of the agitation or of visual hallucinations associated with the withdrawal.

As previously discussed, it is very important not to miss head injuries in this group of patients that are notoriously difficult to assess. If there are signs of a head injury in these patients, brain imaging should be considered.

This patient also has signs of possible encephalopathy and the eye signs (nystagmus) could be related to the excess alcohol but could also be a sign of Wernicke's encephalopathy. He should be treated for possible acute thiamine deficiency in addition to the withdrawal, as this could progress if left untreated, with disastrous results.

Management

This man requires close observation, intravenous thiamine, treatment for alcohol withdrawal (lorazepam/chlordiazepoxide) and a CT scan to exclude intracerebral pathology.

Outcome

His CT/head scan was normal and his agitation and confusion settled with regular thiamine and chlordiazepoxide.

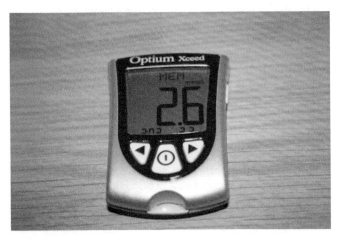

A blood glucose meter.

Further reading

Simon C, Everitt H, Kendrick T. *Oxford Handbook of General Practice*, Second Edition. Oxford University Press, Oxford, 2002.

Tintinalli J, Kelen G, Stapczynski S, *et al. Emergency Medicine: A Comprehensive Study Guide.* Sixth Edition. McGraw-Hill, New York, 2003.

Wyatt JP, Illingworth R, Graham C, *et al. Oxford Handbook of Emergency Medicine,* Third Edition. Oxford University Press, Oxford, 2006.

CHAPTER 13

The Shocked Patient

Arun Chaudhuri

CASE HISTORY

A 68-year-old woman rapidly develops severe breathlessness, clamminess and agitation. She was well 2 days ago, when a non-productive cough and a fever began. The symptoms have progressed since then and become much worse today with intermittent drowsiness and mottling of her skin. She has no chest pain or wheeze, but her husband noticed she has not passed much urine lately and that she looks much paler today with cold hands and feet. She consulted her GP yesterday who thought she had a viral upper respiratory tract infection. She took some over-the-counter 'flu' remedy tablets this morning. She has a past history of ischaemic heart disease, hypertension and type 2 diabetes mellitus. She has never smoked and there is no history of chronic obstructive airway disease or bronchial asthma. Recently she enjoyed a wonderful holiday in Greece and returned 3 days ago. Her medication includes aspirin, bisoprolol, isosorbide mononitrate SR, irbesartan, gliclazide and metformin. She is a retired nurse and lives independently with her husband.

Question: What differential diagnosis would you consider from the history?

Shock arises from an inadequate flow of blood to organs and tissues: the result is organ dysfunction (see Figure 13.1 and Box 13.1). There are three broad types of shock (see Box 13.2) from which four subtypes merit careful consideration in this case.

Septic shock

This form of shock is caused by the systemic response to a severe infection. Identifying the systemic response (systemic inflammatory response syndrome: SIRS) is extremely important so that appropriate management can be started early: all frontline healthcare professionals should be familiar with diagnosing sepsis (see Box 13.3).

Septic shock occurs most frequently in elderly (≥65 years), immunocompromised patients, or those who have undergone an invasive procedure in which there is high chance of bacteraemia. Infection of the lungs, abdomen or urinary tract is most common. Micro-organisms such as Gram-positive and Gram-negative

bacteria, viruses, fungi, rickettsiae and protozoa can all produce septic shock. Systemic infection and toxins released by the infectious organisms produce interleukins leading to metabolic and circulatory derangement.

Haemodynamic changes in septic shock occur in two characteristic patterns: early or hyperdynamic, and late or hypodynamic septic shock. In hyperdynamic septic shock the extremities are usually warm. Total oxygen delivery may be increased while oxygen extraction is reduced leading to cellular hypoxia. As sepsis progresses, hypodynamic shock develops leading to vasoconstriction and reduced cardiac output. The patient usually becomes markedly breathless, febrile and sweaty with cool, mottled and often cyanotic peripheries. Multiple organ failure develops with a striking increase in serum lactate. The mortality from septic shock remains staggeringly high; approximately 35–40% of patients die within 1 month of onset of septic shock.

Hypovolaemic shock

This most common form of shock, results either from the loss of red blood cell mass and plasma from haemorrhage or from loss of plasma volume alone arising from extravascular fluid sequestration or gastrointestinal, urinary and insensible losses. Hypovolaemic shock is usually diagnosed easily if the source of volume loss is obvious, but the diagnosis can be extremely difficult if the source is occult, such as into the gastrointestinal tract. In the latter case, a history of non-steroidal anti-inflammatory use, dark sticky stool (melaena), and upper abdominal pain is helpful. A rectal examination is mandatory to detect occult melaena.

Mild hypovolaemia (≤15% loss of the blood volume) produces mild tachycardia without any external signs, especially in a supine resting adult patient. With moderate hypovolaemia (loss of 15–30% of blood volume) the patient will have significant postural hypotension and tachycardia despite normal supine blood pressure, although the pulse pressure will be reduced.

Classic signs of shock appear if hypovolaemia is severe (≥30% loss of the blood volume). The patient develops marked tachycardia, supine hypotension, oliguria, and agitation or confusion, progressing to coma. The transition from mild to severe hypovolaemic shock can be insidious or extremely rapid. If severe shock is not reversed rapidly, especially in elderly patients and those with multiple comorbidities, it can lead to ischaemic injury and to irreversible decline.

ABC of Emergency Differential Diagnosis. Edited by F. Morris and A. Fletcher.
© 2009 Blackwell Publishing, ISBN: 978-1-4051-7063-5.

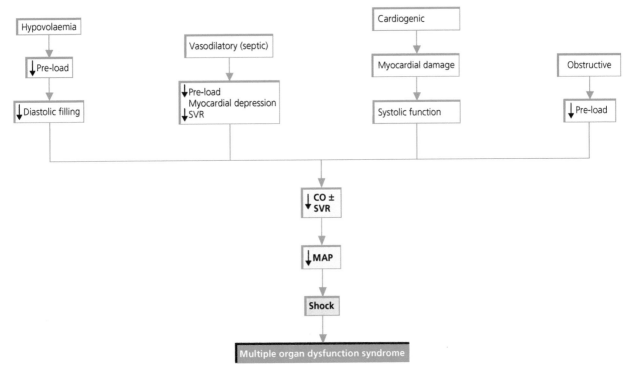

Figure 13.1 Flowchart showing the development of multiple organ dysfunction syndrome. CO, cardiac output; MAP, mean arterial pressure; SVR, systemic vascular resistance.

Box 13.1 **Features common to different varieties of shock**

- **Hypotension**
  - ○ Systolic BP <90 mmHg or
  - ○ Drop in systolic blood pressure of >40 mmHg
  - ○ Profound refractory hypotension in the late stage of shock
- **Cool, clammy skin: except in vasodilatory shock**
- **Signs of hypovolaemia:** oliguria, tachycardia, orthostatic hypotension, poor skin turgor, absent axillary sweat and dry mucous membranes
- **Change in mental state:** agitation, confusion, delirium and ending in obtundation or frank coma
- **Metabolic acidosis:** due to increased lactate production

Cardiogenic shock

Cardiogenic shock is a state of inadequate tissue perfusion due to cardiac dysfunction. It occurs most commonly as a complication of acute myocardial infarction, but it may also be seen in patients with severe tachy- or bradyarrhythmias, valvular heart disease or in the terminal stage of chronic heart failure of any cause, including ischaemic heart disease and dilated cardiomyopathy.

Cardiogenic shock complicates 6–9% of acute myocardial infarction (MI). The majority of patients have ST-elevation MI (STEMI), but cardiogenic shock can also occur in patients with a non-ST elevation acute coronary syndrome. In establishing the diagnosis, a history of cardiac disease or MI is helpful, along with associated physical findings of haemodynamic instability,

peripheral vasoconstriction and pulmonary and/or systemic venous congestion. An ECG is essential and a normal tracing almost rules out shock of cardiac origin.

In compressive or obstructive cardiogenic shock, the heart and surrounding structures are less compliant and despite normal filling pressures there is inadequate diastolic filling. Clinical features of massive pulmonary embolism (chest pain, collapse, evidence of DVT), or pericardial tamponade (penetrating thoracic injury, raised JVP, muffled heart sounds, impalpable apex beat) may be present, but any cause of increased intrathoracic pressure such as tension pneumothorax or excessive positive pressure ventilation can also cause compressive cardiogenic shock.

Anaphylactic shock

Anaphylaxis is a serious allergic reaction that is rapid in onset (usually less than an hour) and may cause death. It is an IgE-mediated, immediate hypersensitivity reaction to proteins (allergens). Anaphylactoid reactions are clinically indistinguishable but are not IgE mediated. The most common causes of anaphylaxis in adults are drugs, such as beta-lactam antibiotics (including penicillins) and non-steroidal anti-inflammatories, foods (seafood, fish and peanuts), insect stings/bites, radiocontrast agents, latex and immunotherapy drugs. No specific trigger can be identified in up to 60% of cases.

Anaphylactic shock occurs in 30% of all cases. Cardiovascular collapse results from increased vascular permeability causing severe hypovolaemia, a reduction in peripheral vascular resistance, and myocardial depression.

Box 13.2 **Types of shock**

1 *Vasodilatory shock*: due to severe decrease in systemic vascular resistance (SVR), often associated with increased cardiac output (CO)
   - Septic shock
   - Anaphylactic shock
   - Neurogenic shock
   - Toxic shock syndrome
   - Adrenal (Addisonian) crisis
   - Myxoedema coma
   - Thyroid storm
   - Drug or toxin reactions, e.g. transfusion reaction, insect bites
   - Activation of the systemic inflammatory response, e.g. pancreatitis, burns

2 *Hypovolaemic shock:* due to decrease in preload leading to reduced cardiac output
   - Fluid loss, e.g. vomiting, diarrhoea, polyuria, burns, pancreatitis, post- operatively, intestinal obstruction and thermal injury
   - Haemorrhage, e.g. gastrointestinal bleeding, fractures, trauma, ruptured aortic aneurysm

3 *Cardiogenic shock:* due to decreased cardiac output

   A Intrinsic
   - Myopathic, e.g. acute myocardial infarction involving more than 40% of left ventricular myocardium, dilated cardiomyopathy, right ventricular infarction
   - Arrhythmias, both tachy- and bradyarrhythmias
   - Mechanical, e.g. acute mitral regurgitation, acute aortic regurgitation in type A aortic dissection, critical aortic stenosis, ventricular septal defect, ruptured ventricular aneurysm

   B Compressive/obstructive
   - Tension pneumothorax
   - Massive pulmonary embolism
   - Cardiac tamponade
   - Severe constrictive pericarditis

Box 13.3 **Sepsis definitions and clinical features**

Systemic inflammatory response syndrome (SIRS) includes two or more of:
- Temperature >38°C or <36°C
- Heart rate >90 beats/minute unless patient is taking medication to reduce the rate (beta blocker or calcium channel blocker) or the heart is paced
- Respiratory rate >20 breaths/minute or mechanically ventilated
- Leucocyte count >12 or <4

Sepsis: presence or presumed presence of an infection accompanied by evidence of SIRS

Severe sepsis: presence of sepsis and at least one of the following signs of organ hypoperfusion or organ dysfunction
- Organ hypoperfusion
  - Increased blood lactate >2 mmol/l
  - Oliguria <0.5 ml/kg/h for at least 1 hour
  - Abnormal peripheral circulation, such as poor capillary refill, mottled skin
  - Acute alteration in mental status
- Organ dysfunction
  - The haematological system, e.g. thrombocytopenia, disseminated intravascular coagulation
  - The pulmonary system, e.g. acute lung injury, acute respiratory distress syndrome
  - The renal system, e.g. acute renal failure
  - The gastrointestinal system with hepatic dysfunction, e.g. ileus, hyperbilirubinaemia (shock liver)
  - The central nervous system, e.g. confusion, delirium
  - Metabolic, e.g. hyperglycaemia, hypoglycaemia (late)

Septic shock: presence of sepsis with refractory hypotension
- Systolic blood pressure <90 mmHg
- A mean arterial pressure <65 mmHg or a 40 mmHg drop in systolic blood pressure compared with baseline
- No response to fluid challenge of 20 ml/kg colloid or 40 ml/kg crystalloid
- Vasopressor dependency after adequate volume resuscitation

The diagnosis of anaphylaxis is clinical but it is often under-diagnosed and undertreated. Most common signs and symptoms are urticaria, angioedema, pruritus and flushing. Danger signs are rapid progression of symptoms, stridor, respiratory distress (e.g. wheezing, constant dry cough), hypotension, dysrhythmia and syncope. The first and the most important therapy of anaphylaxis is intramuscular epinephrine, and many patients carry an Epipen® if they know they are at risk.

Other causes of shock not suggested by the history

Neurogenic shock
Neurogenic shock results from the interruption of sympathetic vasomotor input after a high cervical spinal cord injury, inadvertent cephalad migration of spinal anaesthesia, or severe head injury. Venodilation occurs in addition to arteriolar dilation, leading to decreased venous return and cardiac output. The extremities are often warm. There may be clinical clues on examination, such as a relative bradycardia, diaphragmatic breathing, and a failure to respond to initial fluid resuscitation.

Pancreatitis
This is usually due to alcohol or a gallstone, but can occur after direct injury or some drugs. There is upper or generalised abdominal tenderness along with features of hypovolaemic shock.

Toxic shock syndrome
This is usually due to the systemic effects of *Staphylococcus aureus* toxin. There is often a history of staphylococcal infection or tampon retention (causing vaginal discharge). There is usually a high fever (40°C), headache, abdominal pain and a confluent red rash. Less commonly, Group A *Streptococcus* causes invasive disease that is complicated by toxic shock syndrome.

Case history revisited

To diagnose anaphylaxis, a history of previous reactions would be useful, and it is important to establish the exact nature and timing of the over-the-counter tablets she took. Along with this, a history of rash and itching would help. The absence of wheeze or chest pain does not suggest anaphylaxis and also common causes of cardiogenic shock, but her history of ischaemic heart disease and recent travel is still important. We need more information about her recent bowel habit, specifically for melaena, to explore the possibility of haemorrhage. Questions tailored to identify recent fever and a source of infection are essential pointers to diagnosing septic shock.

Examination

She is distressed with mild confusion. There is no rash, and she has cool, mottled peripheries. Observations are respiratory rate 40 breaths/minute, heart rate 110/minute, oxygen saturation 88% breathing air, temperature 35.8°C, blood pressure 80/60 mmHg. She has passed minimal urine.

Jugular venous pressure is not elevated and peripheral oedema is absent. There is no calf swelling or tenderness suggesting deep vein thrombosis. Heart sounds are normal without any added sound and there is no parasternal heave. Chest examination reveals right basal crackles without wheeze. Abdominal examination is unremarkable and rectal examination normal.

Question: Given the history and examination findings what is your principal working diagnosis?

Principal working diagnosis – septic shock

There is ample evidence of organ dysfunction and poor blood flow, so shock is confirmed. Sepsis is promoted by evidence

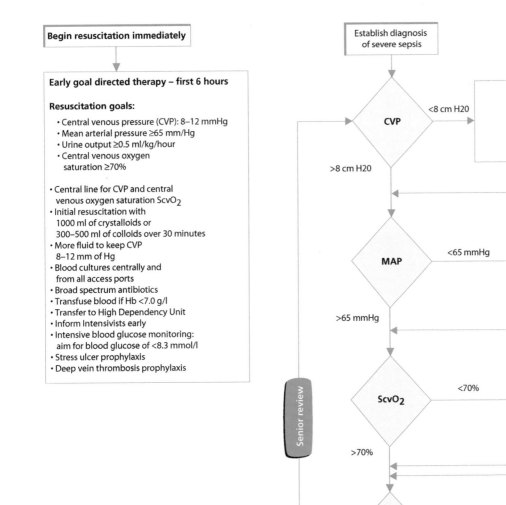

Figure 13.2 Management of severe sepsis and septic shock: hypotension or serum lactate >4 mmol/l.

of hypovolaemia, signs of a respiratory infection, and the history and examination findings that steer away from other differentials. In particular, there are no signs of cardiogenic or obstructive shock here. The absence of wheeze or an urticarial rash make anaphylaxis very unlikely, and the absence of obvious or occult haemorrhage makes haemorrhagic shock less likely (but still possible).

Management

Resuscitation is essential. Oxygen, secure wide bore intravenous access and fluid resuscitation should be simultaneous with investigation. Blood tests including blood cultures are mandatory, as are an ECG, chest X-ray and urinalysis (plus a catheter). Early senior clinical involvement, often with critical care support is necessary to ensure the correct diagnosis and treatments are secured.

Severe sepsis and septic shock are major healthcare problems, affecting millions of individuals around the world every year, killing one in four and often more in the developing and underdeveloped world. Appropriate interventions administered within the first few hours after severe sepsis develops influence the outcome (see Figure 13.2).

Discussion of specific interventions for other causes of shock is beyond the scope of this chapter.

Outcome

Our patient failed to respond to two fluid challenges and required treatment in a high dependency unit with antibiotics and inotropic vasoconstrictors. This was sufficient to ward off the need for dialysis as she recovered slowly from her pneumonia over the following 10 days.

Further reading

Annane D, Bellissant E, Carvallion JM. Septic shock. *Lancet* 2005; **365**: 63–78.

Dellinger RP, Levy MM, Carlet JM, *et al.* Surviving Sepsis Campaign: international guidelines for management of severe sepsis and septic shock: 2008. *Critical Care Medicine* 2008; **36**:296–327.

Hotchkiss RS, Karl IE. The pathophysiology and treatment of shock. *New England Journal of Medicine* 2003; **348**:138–150.

Kortgen A, Niederprum P, Bauer M. Implementation of an evidence-based 'standard operating procedure' and outcome in septic shock. *Critical Care Medicine* 2006; **34**:943–949.

Magder S. Central venous pressure: a useful but not so simple measurement. *Critical Care Medicine* 2006; **34**:2224–2227.

Nguyen HB, Corbett SW, Steel R, *et al.* Implementation of a bundle of quality indicators for the early management of severe sepsis and septic shock is associated with decreased mortality. *Critical Care Medicine* 2007; **35**: 1105–1112.

Ramrakha P, Moore K. *Oxford Handbook of Acute Medicine*, Second Edition. Oxford University Press, Oxford, 2004.

Rivers E, Nguyen B, Havstad S, *et al.* Early goal-directed therapy in the treatment of severe sepsis and septic shock. *New England Journal of Medicine* 2001; **345**:1368–1377.

SAFE Study Investigators. A comparison of albumin and saline for fluid resuscitation in the intensive care unit. *New England Journal of Medicine* 2004; **350**:2247–2256.

Shapiro NI, Howell MD, Talmor D, *et al.* Implementation and outcomes of the Multiple Urgent Sepsis Therapies (MUST) protocol. *Critical Care Medicine* 2006; **34**:1025–1032.

Shorr AF, Micek ST, Jackson WL Jr, *et al.* Economic implementation of an evidence based sepsis protocol: can we improve outcomes and lower costs? *Critical Care Medicine* 2007; **35**:1257–1262.

Tintinalli J, Kelen G, Stapczynski S, *et al. Emergency Medicine: A Comprehensive Study Guide*, Sixth Edition. McGraw-Hill, New York, 2003.

Wyatt JP, Illingworth R, Graham C, *et al. Oxford Handbook of Emergency Medicine*, Third Edition. Oxford University Press, Oxford, 2006.

CHAPTER 14

Palpitations

Charles Heatley

CASE HISTORY

A 32-year-old woman presents with a 4-week history of 'palpitations' which have been increasing in frequency and now occur several times each day, making her increasingly anxious. She is also complaining of episodic 'thumping' feelings in her chest as if her heart is 'trying to escape from her chest'. She has managed to keep working as a cleaner and caring for her two children, involving a half mile walk uphill to school each day. She drinks little alcohol, does not smoke, and consumes six cups of coffee daily. She has no significant past medical history although she has lost over a stone in weight in the last 3 months without dieting. She is on a combined oral contraceptive.

Question: What differential diagnosis would you consider from the history?

'Palpitations' describes the awareness of one's heart beating, usually because the beats are more forceful, faster or irregular than normal. It is a disturbing symptom for patients but does not usually represent any structural abnormality of the heart and is not commonly a life-threatening condition.

Careful questioning can usually identify normal sensations in a healthy patient and the presence of significant arrhythmia. Ask the patient about the pattern of each event. An open question such as, 'Can you describe what you mean by palpitations?' will give the patient an opportunity to describe the episode in more detail. Further important questions appear in Box 14.2, and associated symptoms in Box 14.3.

The differential diagnosis will include increased awareness of the heartbeat, an arrhythmia, panic attacks and thyrotoxicosis.

Increased awareness

Some patients become aware of their normal heart beat which they find unpleasant. This may occur when they are relaxing in a quiet environment, or be provoked by exercise or emotional upset. Stimulants such as alcohol, tobacco and ephedrine may also provoke this problem (see Box 14.4). Increased awareness of premature beats can lead to a feeling that the heart has missed/skipped a beat

---

Box 14.1 **Causes of palpitations**

- Sinus tachycardia
- Premature beats
- Narrow complex tachycardias:
  ○ Paroxysmal supraventricular tachycardia
  ○ Atrial fibrillation/flutter
- Broad complex tachycardia
- Ventricular tachycardia

Box 14.2 **Important questions about palpitations**

- The duration of each attack
- Whether there is an abrupt or gradual onset
- Whether the rhythm is regular or irregular
- At what rate the patient perceives the heart is beating
- Whether attacks occur at rest or on exertion
- Accompanying symptoms – breathlessness, chest pain
- Estimate coffee and alcohol intake
- Other symptoms, e.g. weight loss, diarrhoea, flushing

Box 14.3 **Symptoms associated with palpitations**

In order of increasing severity and decreasing frequency:
- None
- Awareness of heart beating
- Missed beats or thumps
- Fatigue, light-headedness, dyspnoea, polyuria (SVT)
- Syncope
- Cardiac arrest

---

and patients worry about the prolonged pause or the 'thump' of the stronger next sinus beat.

Arrhythmias (see Box 14.1)

Narrow complex tachycardia

Those tachycardias arising from the atria or the atrioventricular node will be conducted to the ventricles in a normal fashion and so will have a normal QRS morphology with a duration of less than 0.12 seconds.

ABC of Emergency Differential Diagnosis. Edited by F. Morris and A. Fletcher.
© 2009 Blackwell Publishing, ISBN: 978-1-4051-7063-5.

The commonest example of this type of arrhythmia is a paroxysmal supraventricular tachycardia. This form of rhythm disturbance occurs in patients with structurally normal hearts and results from a 'short circuit' in the wiring system. These tachycardias start and finish abruptly and may last for seconds, minutes, hours or days. The heart rate is usually between 150 and 250 beats/minute, is regular, and is usually well tolerated by the patient.

Less common forms of narrow complex tachycardias include atrial tachycardia.

Atrial fibrillation and atrial flutter

In contrast to PSVT, these rhythm disturbances are usually associated with heart disease, e.g. hypertension, ischaemic and valvular heart disease and alcohol.

In atrial fibrillation the atrial rate is extremely rapid at 600/minute, with a variable degree of atrioventricular block resulting in a ventricular rhythm that is *irregular* and bears no relationship to the atrial rhythm. Atrial fibrillation can be paroxysmal, persistent or permanent; the longer it has been present, the longer it is likely to persist (see Figure 14.1).

Atrial flutter, which is much less common than fibrillation, is characterised by a rapid atrial rate at 300/minute with variable conduction through the atrioventricular node, resulting in a slower ventricular response. The ECG is usually characterised by a 'saw toothed' pattern of P wave activity.

Ventricular tachycardia

Whilst occasional or frequent single ventricular ectopics are a common finding, ventricular tachycardia is defined as three or more consecutive ventricular beats at a rate of 120 beats/minute or more. It is called sustained if the ventricular tachycardia persists for 30 seconds or more. Although it is more commonly associated with structural heart disease than other arrhythmias, it can still occur in a healthy heart.

Fast ventricular rates in association with heart disease are more likely to give rise to symptoms. The ECG shows complexes greater than 0.12 seconds in duration.

The identification of ventricular tachycardia demands prompt further investigation in secondary care, as ventricular tachycardia can lead to ventricular fibrillation (see Figure 14.2).

Panic attack

Patients suffering from anxiety frequently present with palpitations associated with a variety of other physical symptoms. Ask whether the patient is anxious about these attacks, experiences anxiety during the attacks or is anxious in general. Commonly patients become more vigilant about the activity of their heart if they are scared about heart disease, particularly if a close friend or family member has recently experienced significant heart problems. There is a specific set of symptoms, thoughts and feelings defining panic attacks which can lead to a positive diagnosis of this disorder (see Box 14.5).

Thyrotoxicosis

Palpitations can occur in association with thyrotoxicosis as sinus tachycardia and atrial fibrillation are commonly recognised in this condition. There are many other symptoms and signs characteristic of this condition (see Box 14.6).

Although palpitations alone are unlikely to be the presenting feature of thyrotoxicosis the diagnosis should be considered in this woman as she has had significant weight loss.

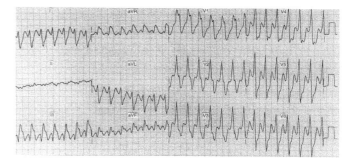

Figure 14.2 Ventricular tachycardia.

Box 14.4 **Drugs/stimulants giving rise to palpitations**

- Caffeine
- Nicotine
- Ephedrine, pseudoephedrine
- Cocaine and crack, amphetamines
- Methylphenidate
- Salbutamol and other inhaled β_2 agonists

Box 14.5 **DSM IV criteria for diagnosing a panic attack**

A discrete period of intense fear or discomfort, in which four (or more) of the following symptoms develop abruptly and reached a peak within 10 minutes:
- Palpitations, pounding heart, or accelerated heart rate
- Sweating
- Trembling or shaking
- Sensations of shortness of breath or smothering
- Feeling of choking
- Chest pain or discomfort
- Nausea or abdominal distress
- Feeling dizzy, unsteady, light-headed, or faint
- Derealization (feelings of unreality) or depersonalization (being detached from oneself)
- Fear of losing control or going crazy
- Fear of dying
- Paresthesias (numbness or tingling sensations)
- Chills or hot flushes

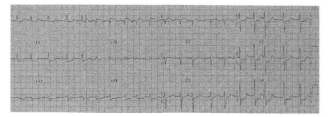

Figure 14.1 Atrial fibrillation.

Case history revisited

On further questioning this woman has two forms of palpitations. The first are episodes of fast regular palpitations with an abrupt onset, lasting for a few minutes at a time, and the second an occasional 'thumping' in her chest, lasting seconds.

There was no history of any other symptoms suggestive of thyrotoxicosis or the use of other stimulants.

Examination

Examination was normal. Her resting heart rate was 76 beats/minute, blood pressure 110/75 mmHg and cardiovascular examination was normal. There were no signs of thyrotoxicosis. The electrocardiogram was normal.

Question: Given the history and examination findings what is your principal working diagnosis?

Principle working diagnosis – Paroxysmal supraventricular tachycardia and premature beats

Management

In many cases a thorough history, examination and electrocardiogram will be all that is required to reassure a patient who is experiencing increased awareness of ventricular ectopics or their normal rhythm.

Appropriate blood tests should be performed to assess thyroid status, urea and electrolytes, liver function and full blood count.

More detailed investigations including 24-hour Holter monitoring, loop event recorders and electrophysiological studies are required in those patients with a clear history suggestive of an arrhythmia.

24-hour Holter monitoring

In this investigation a patient has a two or three lead ECG machine fitted. This is portable and can be comfortably worn for 24 hours during which the patient is asked to complete a diary documenting any symptomatic episodes that may correlate with recorded ECG abnormalities. These machines can later be interrogated by computer resulting in a report documenting episodes of abnormal rhythm and thereafter confirmed by a cardiac technician or cardiologist. The advantage of this investigation is that a complete record is obtained over 24 hours and can correlate symptoms with either normal or abnormal rhythm problems. The disadvantage is in patients whose symptoms are less frequent in which case repeated or sometimes prolonged investigation is required.

Loop event recorders

A loop event recorder can be worn for 2–3 weeks. It is a smaller unit which continuously monitors rhythm but only records to memory on activation by the patient during symptomatic episodes, from 1 minute before to 1 minute after activation. The rhythm strips are later analysed and reported.

Outcome

Twenty-four hour Holter monitoring revealed that this woman was experiencing frequent ventricular ectopics only. All her symptoms settled once she stopped drinking coffee.

Further reading

Ramrakha P, Moore K. *Oxford Handbook of Acute Medicine*, Second Edition. Oxford University Press, Oxford, 2004.

Simon C, Everitt H, Kendrick T. *Oxford Handbook of General Practice*, Second Edition. Oxford University Press, Oxford, 2002.

Swanton RH. *Cardiology*, Fifth Edition. Blackwell Publishing, Oxford, 2003.

Tintinalli J, Kelen G, Stapczynski S, *et al. Emergency Medicine: A Comprehensive Study Guide*, Sixth Edition. McGraw-Hill, New York, 2003.

Warrell DA, Cox TM, Firth JD, Benz EJ Jr (Eds). *Oxford Textbook of Medicine*, Fourth Edition. Oxford University Press, Oxford, 2003.

Wyatt JP, Illingworth R, Graham C, *et al. Oxford Handbook of Emergency Medicine*, Third Edition. Oxford University Press, Oxford, 2006.

CHAPTER 15

Low Back Pain

Richard Kendall

CASE HISTORY

A 62-year-old retired teacher complains of back pain. The pain is situated in his lower back and started fairly abruptly this morning. He fell backwards getting out of the bath 2 days previously and feels that the pain is possibly related to the fall, although yesterday he was fully mobile and pain free. The pain is constant and moderately severe scoring 6/10. It is localised slightly to the left of his lumbar region and is not made particularly worse by movement. He has also experienced some abdominal discomfort. He has no new urinary symptoms and his bowels are also normal. He has tried taking some paracetamol and codeine for the pain but it has not helped. His past history includes ulcerative colitis and benign prostatic hypertrophy. His current medication is prednisolone 5 mg and mesalazine 500 mg three times a day.

Question: What differential diagnosis would you consider from the history?

Low back pain has a very wide differential ranging from the life threatening to the 'common or garden' (see Box 15.1). It is important to be methodical in your approach and consider all relevant diagnoses, especially those that are more serious (see Table 15.1).

Mechanical back pain

The vast majority of the population have experienced mechanical low back pain at some stage in their lives. This is the commonest cause of back pain. Mechanical back pain is a heterogeneous group of pathologies relating to the vertebral column and associated soft tissues.

Degenerative disease of the intervertebral discs and facet joints can cause pain as can damage to the ligaments or adjacent muscles (paravertebral muscles). The exact nature of the problem is not important since the treatment of mechanical back pain is the same whatever the specific cause. The key is to be comfortable with the diagnosis and to ensure that no 'red flag' symptoms are present suggesting serious causes of back pain. Typically there is a history of recurrent backache and stiffness which is provoked by an activity such as exercise, digging or lifting. In addition there is commonly back stiffness especially in the morning and after sitting still.

ABC of Emergency Differential Diagnosis. Edited by F. Morris and A. Fletcher.
© 2009 Blackwell Publishing, ISBN: 978-1-4051-7063-5.

Box 15.1 Differential diagnosis for low back pain

Common causes:
- Mechanical back pain
- Fractured vertebrae – direct trauma/osteoporotic
- Prolapsed intervertebral disc
- Renal colic
- Pyelonephritis

Less common causes:
- Bony malignancy – secondary infiltration (lung, breast, prostate, renal, thyroid cancer)
- Multiple myeloma
- Symptomatic aortic aneurysm (either stretching or ruptured)
- Pancreatitis

Rare but important causes:
- Discitis or osteomyelitis
- Epidural abscess
- Prostatitis
- Retroperitoneal tumours–pancreatic carcinoma, sarcoma

Table 15.1 Low back pain: red flag symptoms.

Red flag symptom	Possible pathology
Saddle area paraesthesia	Cauda equina syndrome
Urinary symptoms such as retention, difficulty passing urine and Incontinence	Cauda equina syndrome
Faecal incontinence	Cauda equina syndrome
Constant pain, at night and rest	Malignant disease or infective process
Fever	Infective process
Abdominal pain	Aortic aneurysm
Sudden onset or cardiovascular collapse	Aortic aneurysm
Trauma	Fracture

Treatment involves gentle mobilisation, simple analgesia and antispasmodics. A combination of paracetamol, low dose diazepam and a NSAID is commonly sufficient. Back exercises and, in those patients with persistent symptoms, physiotherapy may be helpful.

Vertebral fracture

This always needs to be considered in patients where there is a history of trauma and in those at risk of osteoporosis. If there is a delay between the injury and onset of pain it is likely the pain is related to a soft tissue injury or an exacerbation of a degenerative condition rather than a fracture. Where there is a convincing history of injury or bony tenderness, plain radiographs of the lumbar spine are indicated. An osteoporotic fracture can occur with minimal or even no trauma and needs to be considered in anyone at risk of osteoporosis. This man is at risk of osteoporosis because of the long term use of steroids to control his inflammatory bowel disease.

Prolapsed intervertebral disc

Intervertebral discs degenerate over time and the disc can herniate to press on the associated nerve root (see Figure 15.1). The characteristic symptom of a prolapsed disc is sciatica. Sciatica is a pain that radiates down the posterior aspect of the leg further than the knee and may radiate as far as the ankle or foot. Signs of a nerve entrapment include muscle weakness, loss of sensation, diminished or absent reflexes, and a positive straight leg raise test.

The straight leg raise test involves positioning the patient supine and raising the leg of the patient by flexing the hip whilst maintaining full knee extension (see Figure 15.2). A positive test is where the patient experiences pain radiating down the posterior of the leg as the nerve roots are stretched.

The commonest nerve roots affected are the L5 nerve from compression of a degenerative L4/L5 disc and the S1 nerve from compression of a degenerative L5/S1 disc (see Table 15.2).

Other causes of nerve root compression include spinal stenosis and the cauda equina syndrome. The spinal column ends at the level of the L1/L2 vertebrae and the bundle of nerve fibres that continues in the spinal canal is named the cauda equina. Cauda equina syndrome relates to the compression of the cauda equina most commonly by the central prolapse of an intervertebral disc (see Figure 15.3). Cauda equina syndrome is a true emergency and must be considered in any patient presenting with back pain (see Box 15.2). Typically the patient complains of bilateral leg pain, with limited straight leg raising and there may be bilateral leg weakness and absent reflexes. The development of bladder or bowel dysfunction and paraesthesiae in the saddle distribution indicates the involvement of the sacral nerve roots S2–4 and is a surgical emergency. Nerve root compression of S2–4 gives rise to laxity of anal tone and loss of perianal sensation (see Figure 15.4).

Table 15.2 Signs and symptoms of L5 and S1 nerve compression.

	L5 nerve (L4/L5 disc)	S1 nerve (L5/S1 disc)
Motor weakness	Dorsiflexion of big toe (extensor hallucis longus) and foot	Plantar flexion of big toe and foot
Sensory deficit	Big toe, medial border foot	Lateral border of foot
Reflexes	Variable /no deficit	Ankle reflex diminished

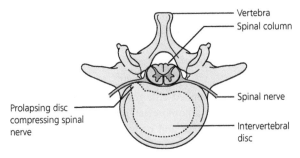

Figure 15.1 Prolapsed disc pressing on associated nerve root.

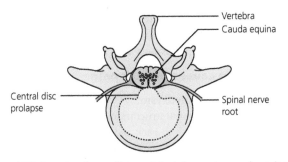

Figure 15.3 Central prolapse of intervertebral disc causing cauda equina syndrome.

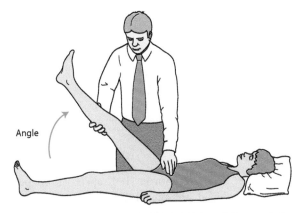

Figure 15.2 Straight leg raising – hip flexed with knee fully extended. Record the maximum angle that the leg is extended from the horizontal position.

Box 15.2 **Symptoms and signs suggestive of cauda equina syndrome**

- Bilateral leg symptoms and/or signs
- Urinary symptoms – retention of urine, difficulty passing urine, incontinence
- Faecal incontinence
- Residual volume of urine after voiding
- Reduced or absent anal tone
- Perianal or perineal paraesthesia

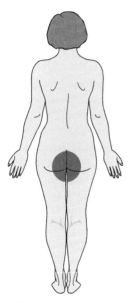

Figure 15.4 Saddle paraesthesiae. Any subjective or objective paraesthesiae in the area shown is suggestive of cauda equina syndrome.

Renal colic

Typically renal colic presents with loin pain that radiates to the groin. On occasions the pain is located only in the loin. There is no history of trauma and the pain characteristically is of sudden onset. Urinary symptoms are common. Microscopic haematuria is present in 95% of cases of renal colic but there are many other causes of microscopic haematuria. Loin tenderness is common but abdominal tenderness is very unusual in renal colic. If there is abdominal tenderness, carefully consider the possibility of an alternative problem, in particular an abdominal aortic aneurysm.

Pyelonephritis

In pyelonephritis the pain and tenderness commonly is located in the loin. There are often lower urinary tract symptoms and associated constitutional symptoms such as fever, rigors and anorexia.

Less common causes of back pain

Symptomatic aortic aneurysm

The aorta is a retroperitoneal structure and typically a symptomatic aortic aneurysm gives rise to back and abdominal pain. Whereas an intraperitoneal rupture of the aorta gives rise to pain of sudden onset and shock, a contained leak may just cause pain. Patients are usually unaware they have an aortic aneurysm. Clinical examination is notoriously unreliable in detecting aortic aneurysms, particularly if the patient is overweight, though the presence of a tender pulsatile expansile mass is highly suggestive. Be wary in patients over the age of 55 who present with apparent renal colic, typically on the left side, as this is a well-recognised presentation of a leaking aneurysm. Occasionally aneurysms that are rapidly growing will be become symptomatic and painful due to the sudden stretching of the arterial wall, but without rupture.

Bony malignancy – metastatic cancer, myeloma

Bony metastases are an important cause to consider in any one with known malignant disease. The five malignancies that most commonly metastasize to bone are lung, prostate, kidney, thyroid and breast. Occasionally bony metastases are the first presentation of underlying malignancy. Bone pain is typically persistent, chronic, unremitting and worse at night. Plain radiographs may not show malignant deposits. If malignant disease is suspected, then a radionucleotide scan (bone scan) is indicated. Myeloma can be difficult to establish and needs to be considered in any person over 60 years with bone pain. Plain radiographs may be normal; a urinary Bence-Jones protein test and plasma electrophoresis are required for diagnosis.

Pancreatitis

Although pancreatitis is relatively common it is unusual for it to present solely with back pain. The pain in pancreatitis is usually located in the upper abdomen and radiates into the back. Serum amylase levels will be elevated, usually seven times greater than normal.

Rare but important causes of back pain

Infective causes – discitis, osteomyelitis, epidural abscess

These conditions are all rare but important to consider in anyone with constitutional symptoms such as fever or rigors and severe back pain. At risk groups are patients where there has been an intervention of some sort (for example a recent nerve root injection), diabetics, injecting drug users and immunosuppressed patients. As with malignancy, the pain associated with infection is persistent and unremitting and often worse at night. On examination there may be localised tenderness and swelling over the affected vertebra. As these conditions are uncommon a high index of suspicion is required which should lead to the full evaluation of any patient in a high risk group who presents with severe non-traumatic back pain.

Prostatitis

Prostatitis is uncommon. At risk groups are those with bladder outflow obstruction and homosexual men. The pain is severe and localised to the lower back and perineum. Prostatic examination is painful with the prostate being exquisitely tender. There may be constitutional features such as fever and rigors. Commonly, there is an associated urinary tract infection.

Case history revisited

Given the differential diagnosis it is important to enquire about urinary symptoms, sphincter disturbance, leg pain and weakness as well as constitutional symptoms. Likewise the examination should include an assessment of the abdomen, urinalysis, the spine, rectal examination and neurology in the lower limbs (see Box 15.3).

Examination

This man's vital signs are normal. He is apyrexial, his pulse is 86 beats/minute, blood pressure 115/85 mmHg and his oxygen saturations are 96% on room air. Abdominal examination reveals an overweight individual with epigastric and left-sided abdominal tenderness. There is no obvious palpable pulsatile mass.

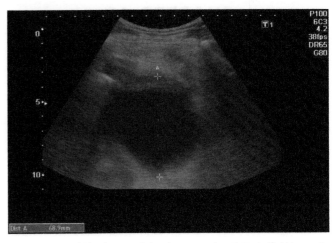

Figure 15.5 Bedside ultrasound showing an aortic aneurysm. Fluid transmits ultrasound and is black on ultrasound images. The aneurysm is the black circular structure in the centre of the picture.

He is minimally tender in the left loin and in the left paravertebral muscles. There is no tenderness along the lumbar spine. Rectal examination is normal, with normal perianal sensation and normal anal tone. His prostate is enlarged but smooth with no tenderness. Neurological examination of his lower limbs is normal with power MRC grade 5/5 in all muscle groups, normal sensation and reflexes. Straight leg raising is to 90° in both legs with no pain. His urinanalysis reveals 1+ of blood but is otherwise normal.

Question: Given the history and examination findings what is your principle working diagnosis?

Principle working diagnosis – possible ruptured aortic aneurysm

In view of the abdominal tenderness and acute onset of pain, a symptomatic aortic aneurysm must be excluded. Renal colic is a possibility but abdominal (as opposed to loin) tenderness is unusual. Microscopic haematuria is in keeping with renal colic but it is unusual to have a first episode of renal colic in your sixties.

He is at risk of osteoporosis due to being prescribed corticosteroids. However, the fact that he was pain free the day after his injury and the lack of bony tenderness, make a fracture unlikely. A mechanical cause for the pain is unlikely since the pain is not made worse by movement.

Outcome

To investigate for an aortic aneurysm, a bedside ultrasound examination of his aorta is undertaken. This shows a 6 cm aortic aneurysm (see Figure 15.5). A CT scan of his abdomen confirms the presence of a 6 cm infra-renal aortic aneurysm with a contained rupture in the left retroperitoneal space. This is repaired and he makes an excellent recovery.

Further reading

Knot A, Polmear A. *Practical General Practice: Guidelines for Effective Clinical Management*, Fourth Edition. Butterworth-Heinemann, Oxford, 2004.

Simon C, Everitt H, Kendrick T. *Oxford Handbook of General Practice*, Second Edition. Oxford University Press, Oxford, 2002.

Tintinalli J, Kelen G, Stapczynski S, *et al. Emergency Medicine: A Comprehensive Study Guide*, Sixth Edition. McGraw-Hill, New York, 2003.

Wardrope J, English B. *Musculo-skeletal Problems in Emergency Medicine*, Oxford University Press, Oxford, 1998.

Wyatt JP, Illingworth R, Graham C, *et al. Oxford Handbook of Emergency Medicine*, Third Edition. Oxford University Press, Oxford, 2006.

Acute Confusion

Steve Goodacre

Question: What differential diagnosis would you consider from the history?

The common pathway for all causes of acute confusion is impaired cerebral function. There are many potential causes (see Table 16.1), therefore a system of classification is useful. A number of causes may co-exist, and an underlying pathology may cause delirium by a variety of mechanisms. For example, pneumonia may cause delirium through hypoxia, hypercapnia, shock, and the toxic effects of sepsis.

A simple system for classifying causes of acute confusion is to divide causes into:
- Lack of vital elements for cerebral function.
- Systemic factors that impair cerebral function.
- Local factors that impair cerebral function.

Hypoglycaemia/hyperglycaemia

Abnormalities of blood glucose should be considered in all cases of delirium, especially if there is a history of diabetes mellitus. Unfortunately, a clear history is often not available and therefore an early assessment of glucose using a bedside meter is essential, as problems are common and easily reversible. Occasionally, a history of missed or changed medication, or recent hypoglycaemic episodes, is available. Patients may be aggressive or behave inappropriately in the early stages, and become progressively drowsy and unconscious as the metabolic problem progresses.

Many patients with hypoglycaemia will be sweaty and clammy. Some will also have a focal neurological sign that resolves when the hypoglycaemia is reversed. Those with hyperglycaemia may be dehydrated and ketoacidotic (see Box 16.1). Hyperglycaemia and hypoglycaemia may be a consequence of other pathology, such as infections, that cause confusion by other mechanisms.

Sepsis

Toxic metabolites and fever can impair cerebral function. This is probably the most common cause of acute confusion in the elderly and may be associated with relatively minor infections, such as chest or urinary tract infection. Patients are usually pyrexial. A careful history often reveals a potential source of infection (e.g. dysuria, cough) and the possibility of meningitis or encephalitis should always be considered. In older people, pneumococcal

Table 16.1 Causes of acute confusion.

Lack of vital elements for brain function	Systemic factors	Local factors
Hypoxia	Renal failure	Infections (meningitis, encephalitis, abscess)
Hyoglycaemia	Hepatic failure	Tumours (primary and secondary)
Shock	Hyperglycaemia	Trauma (concussion, brain injury, intracranial haematoma)
	Drugs (overdose, side effect or withdrawal)	Haemorrhage (subarachnoid or intracerebral)
	Sepsis	Infarction
	Electrolyte disturbance	Epilepsy (post ictal)
	Hypothermia	

Box 16.1 **Clinical features of diabetic ketoacidosis**

- Deep rapid breathing (Kussmaul)
- Tachycardia and shock
- Vomiting
- Abdominal pain
- Drowsiness and confusion
- Dehydration
- Polyuria

ABC of Emergency Differential Diagnosis. Edited by F. Morris and A. Fletcher.
© 2009 Blackwell Publishing, ISBN: 978-1-4051-7063-5.

meningitis often presents with acute confusion, and a history of a recent ear, chest or sinus infection is very relevant. *Listeria* meningitis is suggested by a history of recent contaminated food ingestion and vomiting. A history of bizarre behaviour, headache, seizures, and a mild to moderate fever, points towards encephalitis, which is usually caused by viruses such as *Herpes simplex*, measles or arboviruses. A contact and travel history is mandatory.

A comprehensive physical examination is necessary in all cases of acute delirium. If sepsis is the cause, there may be abdominal tenderness or urinary retention in urinary tract infection, or crackles, tachypnoea and hypoxia in respiratory infection. Signs of meningism, such as neck stiffness, photophobia, papilloedema, or Kernig's sign, can be subtle especially in the elderly.

Stroke/head injury

In the elderly, ischaemic stroke is common and acute confusion often accompanies this if the speech area from an anterior circulation infarction is affected. A history of rapid onset, along with risk factors such as hypertension, hypercholesterolaemia, or diabetes points to stroke, and there is usually a focal neurological deficit if you look carefully. In all age groups subarachnoid or intra-cerebral bleeding can occur spontaneously and, although more typically presenting as severe headache or loss of consciousness, may present as acute confusion.

Concussive head injuries may cause transient disorientation, while intracranial injuries (cerebral contusion, cerebral haematoma, extradural or subdural haematoma) may cause more prolonged confusion that progresses to coma. Trauma may be obvious, but delays in diagnosis are frequent when the patient is intoxicated (acute extradural haematoma) or elderly (chronic subdural haematoma) because external injury is not always obvious. Subdural haematomas can develop after as apparently innocuous a mechanism as a stumble when there is cerebral atrophy and dural veins are vulnerable to tearing.

Other causes of acute delirium not suggested by the history

Lack of vital elements for cerebral function

1 *Hypoxia.* Patients with confusion due to hypoxia are typically agitated, anxious and breathless. Common causes include pneumonia, heart failure, pulmonary embolus and bronchoconstriction.
2 *Shock.* Inadequate circulation leading to inadequate cerebral perfusion. Patients who are shocked are likely to be pale, clammy and have cool peripheries. Low blood pressure is a late sign. Depending upon the cause, the patient may be tachycardic.

Systemic factors that impair cerebral function

1 *Metabolic causes.* Hyponatraemia or hypercalcaemia may present with acute confusion, particularly if the electrolyte disturbance develops rapidly: clinical diagnosis may be difficult with little history. A careful drug history may point to a metabolic cause. High blood urea due to renal failure can cause confusion and uraemia is usually associated with muscular twitching and signs of dehydration.

Patients with hepatic encephalopathy are jaundiced and may have a flapping tremor. Since alcohol is a common cause, patients may also show features of other alcohol-related disorders, such as alcohol withdrawal or delirium tremens.

2 *Drugs.* Routine or excessive use of a wide variety of prescribed drugs can cause patients to become confused, especially the elderly. Drug overdose or intoxication typically causes a depressed conscious level, but some drug effects may present as acute confusion. These might include recreational use of amphetamines, cocaine or LSD, or overdose of tricyclic antidepressants. Patients would be younger than the case presented and would typically be agitated with a rapid pulse and dilated pupils.

Drugs can also cause confusion if they are withdrawn from a dependent patient. The most common occurrence of this sort would be alcohol withdrawal. This is typically associated with coarse tremor, tachycardia, sweating, agitation and occasionally fitting.

3 *Hypothermia.* Young, healthy patients are unlikely to develop hypothermia unless they suffer prolonged exposure to very cold conditions or are immersed in water. In these cases hypothermia is easy to recognise. The diagnosis is more difficult in the elderly, those dependent on alcohol, or those with chronic diseases, who may suffer hypothermia in association with other chronic illness, falls, or poor social conditions.

4 *Pain.* The superimposition of pain onto another medical problem (such as dementia) can lead to a sudden worsening of confusion. A careful history and comprehensive examination should establish if there is an acute injury or an occult painful problem such as peritonitis. Remember to check the hips of elderly patients who have fallen: impacted fractures are common.

Local factors that impair cerebral function

1 *Tumours.* Primary brain tumours and secondary metastases may cause acute confusion through direct cerebral effects or raised intracranial pressure. The diagnosis is suggested by an associated headache that is worse on coughing and straining, and associated vomiting. Frontal tumours may present as unusual behaviour without other symptoms or signs. The onset is usually insidious, however.
2 *Epilepsy.* Following a seizure most patients will undergo a period of confusion as they regain consciousness. This usually resolves within an hour. If it does not resolve then alternative causes should be sought.

Psychiatric causes

Psychiatric illness, almost by definition, does not cause acute confusion states. However, it is important to distinguish between acute confusion due to an organic cause and acute psychosis due to a psychiatric cause. The presence of auditory hallucinations and evidence of thought disorder suggest psychiatric illness.

Case history revisited

Returning to our case, the diagnosis is not clear: many possible differentials could apply. Although it may be difficult to establish, a history of possible drug overdose should be ruled out through a thorough review of medication. A history of transient neurological symptoms or fluctuating confusion recently, points more toward a

Box 16.2 **Hodkinson mental test**

Score one point for each question answered correctly to give total score out of 10
1 Patient's age
2 Time (to nearest hour)
3 Address given, for recall at end of test (42 West Street)
4 Name of hospital (or area of town if at home)
5 Current year
6 Patient's date of birth
7 Current month
8 Years of the First World War
9 Name of monarch (or president)
10 Count backwards from 20 to 1 (no errors allowed but may correct self)

transient ischaemic attack and stroke. If there have been falls, then traumatic brain injury is more likely. Recent dysuria, frequency, cough, or upper respiratory infection may suggest sepsis.

Examination

Our patient is calm and drowsy when left alone, but resists examination, with all limbs moving equally and normally. There is a small bruise to her left temple and her mucous membranes are dry. Observations are temperature 37.8°C, pulse 104 beats/minute, blood pressure 156/80 mmHg, respiratory rate 18/minute, oxygen saturations 96% on air. Blood glucose is 6.8 mmol/l by meter.

The patient scores 0/10 on the Hodkinson mental test (see Box 16.2). Heart sounds are normal, and chest examination reveals a few crackles at both lung bases. There is no peritonism, but there is vague lower abdominal tenderness. A full neurological examination is impossible because of lack of understanding and cooperation, but there is no obvious focal deficit or neck stiffness.

Question: Given the history and examination findings what is your principal working diagnosis?

Principal working diagnosis – Acute delirium due to urinary tract infection (with probable pre-existing cognitive impairment)

The normal glucose level ensures hypoglycaemia is ruled out. The presence of fever makes sepsis much more likely and the lower abdominal tenderness suggests urinary tract infection. Infection in other areas cannot be totally excluded but seem much less likely. Although there is a bruise, head injury is likely to be coincidental, and there is no marked abnormality of conscious level or focal weakness. Nevertheless, this important differential diagnosis still needs consideration.

Management

Management should ultimately be directed at the underlying cause. A systematic approach will ensure that the patient does not suffer avoidable harm while the diagnosis is sought, that unnecessary tests are avoided, and that the correct diagnosis is identified (see Box 16.3).

Box 16.3 **Management of confusion**

ABCDEFG
• Airway, breathing, circulation, don't ever forget glucose
• Treat any problems identified

Clinical history
• Paramedics, friends, relatives and contacts
• Events, previous illnesses, drug use, recent illness or trauma

Clinical examination
• Pulse, BP, oxygen saturation, BM, temperature
• Alert bracelets, personal details, drug use, injuries, sources of infection
• Pupils
• Spontaneous movements, tone and reflexes
• Cardiovascular, respiratory and abdominal examination

Simple tests
• Arterial blood gases
• Full blood count, urea and electrolytes, blood glucose, liver function tests, calcium, thyroid function
• Urinalysis
• Chest X-ray

CT scan of the brain

Lumbar puncture

ABCDEFG

This first crucial step is to assess the Airway, Breathing and Circulation, and then check blood sugar (Don't Ever Forget Glucose). If any problem is identified it should be treated immediately. This will ensure that the patient does not die or suffer brain damage while further investigations are undertaken and will identify if confusion is due to a lack of vital elements for cerebral function.

It is usually most appropriate to start with the simplest investigations and then work up. Our patient ultimately requires a CT scan, but scanning a confused and possibly unstable patient is challenging and potentially risky. If the cause of the confusion can be identified by a simple test then difficult procedures may be avoided.

Blood tests may show evidence of infection or metabolic abnormalities. Urinalysis and chest X-ray are required to identify common sites of infection, but routine drug screening is rarely helpful.

It is often possible to control agitation by providing a calm, quiet and reassuring environment. A number of factors may worsen agitation and disorientation, particularly in the elderly, but may be relatively easy to address. Painful conditions should be treated with appropriate analgesia. Oral fluid intake should be encouraged. Spectacles and hearing aids should be checked to ensure they are in good working order. Sedation should only be used as a last resort and if the patient is at risk of harming themselves.

Outcome

This patient's blood tests revealed evidence of dehydration and infection and a urinalysis positive for nitrites and leucocytes. She settled with intravenous fluids and her family's reassurance. A CT brain scan was normal apart from showing cerebral atrophy.

She was given antibiotics for her urinary tract infection and her delirium settled after 5 days.

Further reading

British Geriatric Society. Guidelines for the Prevention, Diagnosis and Management of Delirium in Older People in Hospital, 2006. **www.bgs.org.uk**/Publications/Clinical%20Guidelines/clinical_1–2_fulldelirium.htm

Brown TM, Boyle MF. ABC of psychological medicine: delirium. Clinical review. *BMJ* 2002; **325**:644–647.

Meagher DJ. Delirium: optimising management. Clinical review. *BMJ* 2001; **322**:144–149.

Patient Plus. Acute Confusional State. www.patient.co.uk/showdoc/40002104/ (accessed 21/09/2007).

Young J, Innouye SK. Delirium in older people. Clinical review. *BMJ* 2007; **334**:842–846.

CHAPTER 17

Shortness of Breath

Kevin Jones and Claire Gardner

Question: What differential diagnosis would you consider from the history?

There are many different causes of shortness of breath, the commonest are listed in Box 17.1.

Box 17.1 **Causes of shortness of breath**

- Asthma
- Chronic obstructive pulmonary disease
- Pulmonary oedema
- Pneumothorax
- Pulmonary embolism
- Pneumonia
- Pleural effusion
- Interstitial lung disease
- Metabolic acidosis
- Hyperventilation
- Anaemia

ABC of Emergency Differential Diagnosis. Edited by F. Morris and A. Fletcher.
© 2009 Blackwell Publishing, ISBN: 978-1-4051-7063-5.

Pneumothorax

A spontaneous pneumothorax should be considered in the differential diagnosis of any patient presenting with acute shortness of breath, particularly if the symptoms came on suddenly (see Figure 17.1). It is important to recognise a pneumothorax promptly as specific treatments can quickly alleviate the patient's symptoms. The story provided by this man is not suggestive of a pneumothorax, which normally presents with sudden onset of shortness of breath associated with pleuritic chest pain. The conditions associated with a pneumothorax are listed in Box 17.2.

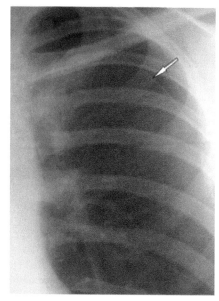

Figure 17.1 Left pneumothorax. Reprinted with permission from *BMJ* 2005; **330**:1493–1497.

Box 17.2 **Conditions associated with pneumothorax**

- Tall, thin male
- Cigarette smoking
- Underlying lung disease most commonly COPD
- Connective tissue disease, e.g. Marfan's

Asthma

This man gives a history of having asthma as a child and when speaking appears to be wheezy. In the last 48 hours he has felt unwell with a persistent cough and chest tightness. This would be entirely in keeping with a respiratory infection precipitating bronchospasm in a susceptible individual. Symptoms are commonly nocturnal, which is also the case with this patient.

Typically an acute exacerbation of asthma is precipitated by a respiratory infection, viral being more common than bacterial. Such an infection may have provoked this episode. Pneumonia is, therefore, a possibility here. This would usually present with cough and sputum (yellow, green or brown) and fever. Supportive features in the history would be pleuritic chest pain, malaise and headache and any history of travel or contacts. The shortness of breath would more commonly be of gradual onset but it is possible to become acutely short of breath with pneumonia. The fact he is not coughing any sputum and has no symptoms of fever does not suggest this diagnosis.

Left ventricular failure

This man's symptoms could be the result of pulmonary oedema. Pulmonary oedema presents with acute shortness of breath and patients frequently are wheezy hence the term 'cardiac asthma'. There may be a cough with classically pink, frothy sputum. Patients with acute pulmonary oedema are often grey, 'ashen', have extreme respiratory distress and their skin is frequently cold and wet. These clinical features strongly point to an underlying diagnosis of pulmonary oedema rather than another common cause of shortness of breath, chronic obstructive pulmonary disease, when the patient's skin is typically warm and dry.

This man is diabetic and has a family history of ischaemic heart disease. In addition to these risk factors he has complained of tightness in his chest over the last 48 hours which could have been the result of an acute coronary syndrome. His shortness of breath could therefore be the result of new cardiac damage giving rise to pulmonary oedema.

Diabetic ketoacidosis (DKA)

Type 1 diabetics often lose their glycaemic control when they become unwell which may result in diabetic ketoacidosis. This condition is due to a lack of insulin, which allows the plasma glucose levels to rise, causing an osmotic diuresis resulting in loss of salt and water from the body. Significant fluid losses lead to hypoperfusion resulting in hypotension and shock. Lack of insulin leads to a change in metabolism causing ketone production and acidosis. DKA is frequently precipitated by infection or other intercurrent illness. Patients present in a variety of ways but common features include nausea, vomiting, abdominal pain, polydipsia, polyuria, altered consciousness and coma.

As the body tries to compensate for the developing metabolic acidosis, patients tend to hyperventilate to discharge carbon dioxide. This compensatory hyperventilation (Kussmaul respiration) can be the most obvious clinical feature and may lead to the erroneous diagnosis of a respiratory illness such as pneumonia or asthma.

The absence of chest signs, the smell of ketones on the breath and a bedside glucose estimation will allow the correct diagnosis to be made.

Other causes of shortness of breath not suggested by the history

Pulmonary embolism (PE)

PE may be associated with sudden onset of shortness of breath and in some individuals this is accompanied by wheezing. There is frequently an obvious risk factor for a PE (see Box 17.3). This man has no obvious risk factors and the prodrome of symptoms for the previous 48 hours would not suggest a PE.

Hyperventilation

In anxiety states which can be exacerbated by chronic alcohol excess, patients may present with acute shortness of breath (see Figure 17.2). Such a presentation, however, would be uncommon in a 49-year-old man without a clear history of anxiety or depression and must remain a diagnosis of exclusion.

Box 17.3 **Risk factors for pulmonary embolism**

- Recent surgery
- Immobility
- Previous DVT/PE
- Malignancy
- Pregnancy/puerperium
- Combined oral contraceptive pill/HRT
- Nephrotic syndrome
- Thrombophilia
- Smoking
- Long flight/car journey
- Obesity

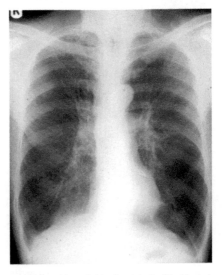

Figure 17.2 Hyperinflated lung fields. Reprinted with permission from *BMJ* 2006; **332**:1261–1263.

Chronic obstructive pulmonary disease

This man's age and the fact that he has never smoked would mitigate against this as a diagnosis and therefore would not form part of the differential diagnosis based upon the history.

Case history revisited

On further questioning this man denies any nausea, vomiting or abdominal pain and is able to confirm that his glycaemic control has been good in the past 48 hours.

He denies any current chest pain or discomfort and reiterates that he simply experienced some intermittent tightness in his chest over the last 48 hours. The cough that he developed has been dry and unproductive.

Examination

On examination he was acutely short of breath with a respiratory rate of 40 breaths/minute. He was pale, clammy, sweaty and cold to touch. His trachea was central and there were no clinical signs of a pneumothorax or any consolidation. Auscultation of his chest revealed widespread wheeze but no crackles. Heart sounds were difficult to hear because of the loud wheezing. His abdomen was soft and there was no evidence of peripheral oedema.

The oxygen saturation probe was reading between 76 and 80% on air and this rose to 90% on high flow oxygen. His pulse was 118 beats/minute and his blood pressure 192/110 mmHg. His peak flow was unrecordable. An electrocardiogram was taken and a chest X-ray was requested (see Figure 17.3). A blood sugar estimation taken at the bedside revealed a glucose level of 15 mmol/l and there was no smell of ketones on his breath. Arterial blood gases showed type one respiratory failure.

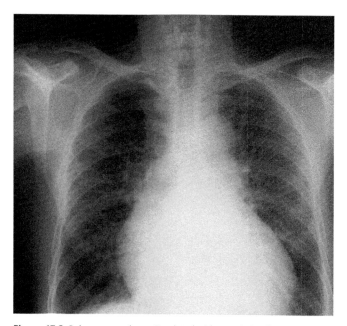

Figure 17.3 Pulmonary oedema. Reprinted with permission from *BMJ* 2000; **320**:297–300.

Given the history and examination findings what is your principle working diagnosis?

Principle working diagnosis – Pulmonary oedema secondary to an acute coronary syndrome in a type 1 diabetic with a family history of ischaemic heart disease

Clinical examination and a chest X-ray rule out pneumothorax. The chest X-ray reveals pulmonary oedema as responsible for his wheeze rather than asthma. His electrocardiogram is abnormal with signs of an ST segment elevation myocardial infarction (STEMI) (see Figure 17.4).

Other clinical signs which point to the diagnosis of acute pulmonary oedema include fine bi-basal crackles and a third heart sound. However, absence of these does not exclude the diagnosis as in this case. The crackles may become more evident as the patient is treated and able to move more air into the smaller airways. A third heart sound is often difficult to hear in a poorly, breathless patient especially if they are wheezy.

His blood sugar is elevated at 15 mmol/l which is not surprising given the myocardial infarction and pulmonary oedema. The absence of ketones on his breath would be against a diagnosis of diabetic ketoacidosis. Not everyone can smell ketones on a patient's breath and it would be important to confirm the absence of ketones with the use of ketone sticks in his urine or blood.

Saturations of 76–80% before oxygen confirm that anxiety-provoked hyperventilation was not the diagnosis.

Management

Oxygen, diuretics and nitrates form the mainstay of treatment of acute pulmonary oedema. The underlying cause must also be addressed; in this case myocardial ischaemia.

This patient should be sat up and provided with a high inspired oxygen concentration. Venous access should be obtained and blood sent for full blood count, urea and electrolytes, cardiac markers, glucose and lipids. Furosemide (50–100 mg) intravenously (i.v.) should be administered slowly.

If the blood pressure is sufficient (systolic >90 mmHg) nitrates can be given, initially in the buccal form, for example, 2 mg buccal glyceryl trinitrate or two puffs of glyceryl trinitrate (GTN) spray. Later an intravenous GTN infusion (1–10 mg/hour) is titrated against blood pressure.

Small doses of intravenous opiates may be useful in some patients as a vasodilator and anxiolytic, e.g. 2.5 mg of morphine. Use this with caution, however, and monitor for any signs of respiratory depression.

Urinary output should be monitored.

Most patients respond quite quickly to these therapies. However, if they are not responding then continuous positive airways pressure (CPAP) can be beneficial. It forces the fluid out of the airways and splints them open, thus improving oxygenation. This should only be used in a patient who can protect their own airway, is cooperative and is not hypotensive (CPAP impairs venous return and may exacerbate hypotension).

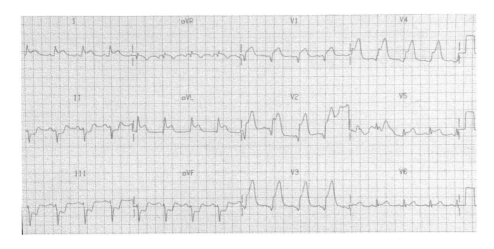

Figure 17.4 Anterior myocardial infection (STEM).

The underlying cause must also be addressed (in this case left ventricular failure due to a myocardial infarction). Given the electrocardiogram and the history it is likely that a myocardial infarction has occurred at some point over the last 48 hours. He has presented too late to be considered for thrombolysis. However, in view of his ongoing pain, ECG changes and pulmonary oedema he should be considered for angiography with a view to angioplasty and coronary stenting. Therefore, a cardiology opinion must be sought. Prior to this aspirin (300 mg) and clopidogrel (600 mg) should be given.

Outcome

This patient's shortness of breath improved with oxygen, diuretics and nitrate infusion. He was seen by a cardiologist who immediately took him to the cardiac catheter laboratory. He had a stent inserted into his left anterior descending artery. He was monitored in hospital for 5 days, started on secondary prevention and discharged on a cardiac rehabilitation programme. His follow-up echocardiogram showed only mild left ventricular impairment.

Further reading

Axford J, O'Callaghan C. *Medicine*, Second Edition. Blackwell Science, Oxford, 2004.

Currie GP (Ed.). *ABC of COPD*. Blackwell Publishing, Oxford, 2007.

Davis RC, Davies MK, Lip GYH. *ABC of Heart Failure*. Blackwell Publishing, Oxford, 2007.

Knot A, Polmear A. *Practical General Practice: Guidelines for Effective Clinical Management*, Fourth Edition. Butterworth-Heinemann, Oxford, 2004.

Ramrakha P, Moore K. *Oxford Handbook of Acute Medicine*, Second Edition. Oxford University Press, Oxford, 2004.

Simon C, Everitt H, Kendrick T. *Oxford Handbook of General Practice*, Second Edition. Oxford University Press, Oxford, 2002.

Tintinalli J, Kelen G, Stapczynski S, *et al. Emergency Medicine: A Comprehensive Study Guide*, Sixth Edition. McGraw-Hill, New York, 2003.

Wyatt JP, Illingworth R, Graham C, *et al. Oxford Handbook of Emergency Medicine*, Third Edition. Oxford University Press, Oxford, 2006.

CHAPTER 18

Collapse of Unknown Cause

Peter Lawson

Question: What differential diagnosis would you consider from the history?

His wife has clearly witnessed a brief episode of transient loss of consciousness (TLOC). The differential diagnosis for this case will be considered, but be aware that this forms part of a wider differential diagnosis for people who are found on the floor at home or who suffer unwitnessed falls or collapse.

A diagnosis of collapse, fall or being found on the floor always indicates the need for a search for the underlying cause (see Figure 18.1). Remember that collapse can occur as part of the presentation of acute medical emergencies without loss of consciousness (e.g. a transient ischaemic attack), with brief loss of consciousness (e.g. myocardial infarction or pulmonary embolism) or with prolonged loss of consciousness (as part of the presentation of an anterior circulation stroke or metabolic coma).

In a clinical situation such as described in the case history, a focused history and examination yields a diagnosis in around 45% of patients, with a 12 lead ECG investigation yielding a diagnosis in a further 5% (see Figure 18.2). The history should include a witness

ABC of Emergency Differential Diagnosis. Edited by F. Morris and A. Fletcher. © 2009 Blackwell Publishing, ISBN: 978-1-4051-7063-5.

report, relevant past medical history, relevant family history and full review of the medication list wherever possible.

Syncope

A useful definition of syncope is a transient, self-limiting loss of consciousness, usually leading to falling. The onset of syncope is relatively rapid, and the subsequent recovery is spontaneous, complete, and usually prompt. The underlying mechanism is a transient global cerebral hypoperfusion (see Brignole *et al.* 2004 for a more detailed discussion of the definition and management).

From this definition it can be seen that syncope is one cause of TLOC but the defining feature is an underlying cardiovascular basis as shown in Box 18.1. It can occur as a single episode or can be recurrent.

The history from the patient is often complemented by that of an eyewitness.

Syncope is suggested by a description of draining of colour from the patient's face, brief unconsciousness and a rapid recovery, usually without confusion. Patients with a vasovagal cause may feel nauseated and unwell for at least several minutes before and/or after the episode. Syncope on exertion or associated with palpitations or chest pain might lead to the search for an arrhythmic cause. Collapse following posture change suggests orthostatic hypotension. Collapse following coughing, swallowing, head turning, defaecation, pain, strong emotion, fear, or prolonged standing suggests neurally mediated reflex syncope.

Past medical and family history can reveal clues of a cardiac cause of syncope through history of cardiac disease (e.g. hypertrophic cardiomyopathy or myocardial infarction) or sudden cardiac death (due, for example, to hypertrophic cardiomyopathy or long QT syndrome).

Examination can help in the differential diagnosis. Pulse rate and rhythm can give evidence of an arrhythmia and bradycardia can persist for minutes to hours after a neurally-mediated collapse. Properly performed lying and standing blood pressure measurement can provide evidence of orthostatic hypotension (see Figure 18.3). Precordial examination can reveal evidence of structural heart disease and causes of left ventricular outflow tract obstruction. Signs include a systolic murmur or abnormality of the apex beat (displacement or character). A full neurological examination is essential.

The prevalence of the causes of syncope depends on the inclusion criteria and population studied. Table 18.1 gives an example.

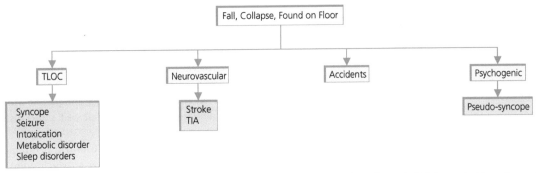

Figure 18.1 Range of mechanisms through which people present with a collapse. TIA, transient ischaemic attack; TLOC, transient loss of consciousness.

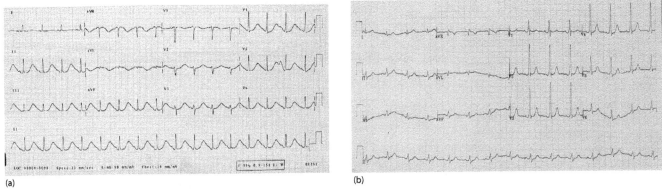

(a)   (b)

Figure 18.2 ECG recordings showing (a) prolonged QT interval and pre-excitation as found in (b) the Wolff–Parkinson–White syndrome.

Box 18.1 **Syncope classification**

Neurally mediated reflex syncope
- Includes vasovagal episodes, carotid sinus syndrome, situational syncope, e.g. micturition

Orthostatic
- e.g. with autonomic failure, volume depletion and medication

Cardiac arrhythmias
- Bradycardia and tachycardia

Structural cardiac or cardiopulmonary disease
- Includes valvular heart disease, obstructive cardiomyopathy and acute conditions such as myocardial infarction and pulmonary embolism

Cerebrovascular
- This is rare, e.g. subclavian steal syndrome

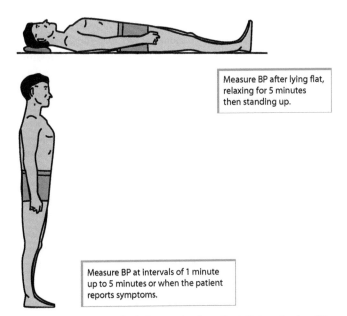

Measure BP after lying flat, relaxing for 5 minutes then standing up.

Measure BP at intervals of 1 minute up to 5 minutes or when the patient reports symptoms.

Figure 18.3 Correct method of measuring for orthostatic hypotension. BP, blood pressure.

Epilepsy

Most forms of epilepsy result in TLOC or a state of altered awareness. An eyewitness account of the events surrounding the attack is very important if it is available. Supportive features in the history include an olfactory or auditory aura, tongue biting, incontinence, tonic and clonic phases, and confusion and drowsiness for more than a few minutes after the attack. However, the presence or absence of any of these features does not conclude or preclude the diagnosis as each may occur as a feature in other causes of TLOC.

The combination of TLOC and jerking will make many witnesses consider that the individual has experienced an epileptic seizure. However, brief jerking is often reported as part of the response to cerebral hypoperfusion and does not necessarily confirm a diagnosis of epilepsy. A clear description of the observed movements

Table 18.1 Final diagnosis in 650 patients presenting to Accident and Emergency with presumed syncope (adapted from Sarasin *et al.* 2001).

Cause of presentation	Number	Percentage
Cardiac	69	11
Arrhythmia	44	(7)
Bradycardia or pause	15	
AV block	15	
Ventricular tachycardia	9	
Supraventricular tachycardia	4	
Acute coronary syndrome	9	
Aortic stenosis	8	
Pulmonary embolism	8	
Non-cardiac	456	70
Vasodepressor syncope	242	(37)
Orthostatic hypotension	158	(24)
Carotid sinus syndrome	6	(1)
Neurological	30	5
Psychiatric	11	1.5
Unknown	92	14
Incomplete evaluation	33	5

and any preceding tonic phase is needed. Post-event confusion, sometimes lasting several minutes, can also be a feature of cerebral hypoperfusion although longer periods of confusion make the chances of underlying epilepsy more likely.

Clinical signs after a seizure are usually confined to injuries sustained during the collapse and subsequent muscle spasms (such as head injury, tongue biting and shoulder dislocation). A full neurological examination is mandatory and may show signs of a focal lesion leading to the seizure or raised intracranial pressure. Sometimes focal weakness or paralysis persists in the post-ictal period (Todd's paresis).

Transient ischaemic attack (TIA)

It is very unusual for a TIA to present with loss of consciousness. If it does, there should be associated neurological signs reflecting posterior circulation ischaemia. These are motor or sensory dysfunction commonly in association with diplopia, dysarthria, ataxia, and/or vertigo. Without these signs, TIA should not appear in the differential diagnosis of someone presenting with a collapse that includes TLOC. The presence or absence of carotid bruits does not help determine the diagnosis and examination for bruits has limited function in the patient presenting with TLOC and no focal neurological signs.

Case history revisited

Reviewing the history, it is likely this man has experienced an episode of syncope. The length of confusion was unhelpful and could have pointed to syncope or a seizure. The arm jerking could also have pointed to a seizure but it was most likely due to cerebral irritation from hypoperfusion. The brief arm weakness was also probably due to cerebral hypoperfusion accentuating the weakness from his previous stroke.

Examination

He looks well and is fully alert. Baseline observations show temperature 36.8°C, pulse 76 beats/minute regular, supine blood pressure 146/80 mmHg, oxygen saturations 98% on air. Heart sounds are normal. A full neurological examination discovered a very mild left arm and leg weakness, compatible with that recorded in his medical notes at a recent clinic visit. Otherwise there were no positive neurological findings.

His blood pressure fell to 120/70 mmHg at 1 minute of standing, and 106/62 mmHg after 3 minutes at which point he mentioned 'dizziness' (which was a light headed sensation rather than a spinning feeling) and feeling 'unwell'.

Immediate investigations

When a patient presents with TLOC a 12 lead ECG is mandatory. Other investigations will be indicated by history and examination and in particular, cardiac enzymes and D-dimers should only be requested if myocardial infarction or pulmonary embolism are strongly suspected.

Question: Given the history and examination findings what is your principal working diagnosis?

Principal working diagnosis – Syncope due to orthostatic hypotension

The history and negative findings on neurological examination point to syncope as the most likely diagnosis. In addition, this man has a substantial fall in blood pressure when he stands. The definition of orthostatic hypotension includes a measured drop of 20 mmHg in systolic BP or 10 mmHg in diastolic BP on standing. This makes orthostatic hypotension the most likely diagnosis in this case, but there now has to be a search for the underlying cause(s) of this drop in blood pressure.

Management

In this case, looking for the cause(s) of orthostatic hypotension requires a thorough review of the medication, level of hydration and any evidence of blood loss, hypoadrenalism or diagnoses associated with autonomic failure.

If the cause of syncope is unclear and the patient has recovered, the next decision is whether he requires admission to hospital. This depends on the risks of recurrence and sudden death, which are determined to a large extent by whether the syncope is cardiac or non-cardiac in origin. The American College of Physicians (ACP) take account of this when they recommend who should be admitted for observation after a syncopal episode (see Box 18.2). Although the period of observation is not stated, overnight ECG monitoring should be sufficient.

Most subsequent investigations can be performed as an outpatient. A 24-hour ECG recording is often performed but it is frequently unrewarding. The use of clinical features improves the diagnostic yield and can focus the use of 24-hour ECG recording on appropriate patients (see Box 18.3).

Box 18.2 **American College of Physicians criteria for hospitalisation after syncope** (taken from Linzer *et al.* 1997)

Definitely hospitalise patients who meet any of the following criteria:

- A history of chest pain
- A past history of coronary artery disease, congestive heart failure, or ventricular arrhythmia
- Physical examination findings of congestive heart failure, valvular disease, or focal neurological deficit
- An electrocardiogram showing ischaemia or infarction*, arrhythmia, long QTc or bundle branch block

Strongly consider hospitalising patients who meet any of the following criteria:

- A history of exertional syncope (in the absence of physical examination evidence of aortic stenosis or other left ventricular outflow obstruction), frequent syncope, or age >70 years
- Physical examination findings of tachycardia, moderate to severe orthostatic changes, or injury
- Suspected cardiac disease

*Most studies excluded non-specific ST and T wave changes

Box 18.3 **Risk of dysrhythmic cause for syncope** (adapted from Sarasin *et al.* 2003)

Risk factors
- Abnormal ECG (excluding non-specific ST and T wave changes)
- History of congestive cardiac failure
- Age >65 years

Numbers of risk factors	Risk of finding dysrhythmia on 24 hour ECG or loop recording
0	0–2%
1	6–17%
2	35–41%
3	27–60%

This information can direct the requesting of 24 hour ECG recordings in people presenting with syncope. Unfortunately no guideline can cover all clinical situations and individual features such as evidence of prolonged QT interval or features of left ventricular outflow obstruction will determine the speed of investigation

If the cause of syncope is unclear the patient should be referred for a specialist opinion on the need for cardiovascular investigations such as tilt table testing and carotid sinus massage to look for neurocardiogenic syncope and carotid sinus syndrome or for more prolonged heart rate and rhythm recording. A CT brain scan is indicated by clinical suspicion of a neurological event. In this case a CT scan is not necessary.

Outcome

This man was admitted to hospital for assessment. His blood tests and ECG were normal. It transpired that his ramipril dose had recently been increased, and his blood pressure settled on resumption of a lower dose.

Question: Can this man be allowed to drive?

This question needs addressing whenever someone presents with loss of consciousness. It is wise always to consult the DVLA Fitness to Drive regulations (www.dvla.gov.uk/media/pdf/medical/aagv1.pdf)

to check the precise wording of each scenario. This man has experienced an explained syncopal episode which should not recur in the sitting position and he is allowed to continue driving.

Further reading

Brignole M, Alboni P, Benditt DG, *et al.* Guidelines on Management (Diagnosis and Treatment) of Syncope – Update 2004. The Task Force on Syncope, European Society of Cardiology. *Europace* 2004; **6**:467–537.

Linzer M, Yang EH, Estes NA III, *et al.* Diagnosing syncope. 1. Value of history, physical examination, and electrocardiography: Clinical Efficacy Assessment Project of the American College of Physicians. *Annals of Internal Medicine* 1997; **126**:989–996.

Linzer M, Yang EH, Estes NA III, *et al.* Diagnosing syncope. 2. Unexplained syncope: Clinical Efficacy Assessment Project of the American College of Physicians. *Annals of Internal Medicine* 1997; **127**:76–86.

Sarasin FP, Louis-Simonet M, Carballo D, *et al.* Prospective evaluation of patients with syncope: a population-based study. *American Journal of Medicine* 2001; **111**:177–184.

Sarasin FP, Hanusa BH, Perneger T, *et al.* A risk score to predict arrhythmias in patients with unexplained syncope. *Academic Emergency Medicine* 2003; **10**:1312–1317.

CHAPTER 19

Abdominal Pain

Suzanne Mason and Alastair Pickering

Question: What differential diagnosis would you consider from the history?

Lower abdominal pain can be considered as the presentation symptom for pathology in two different anatomical 'systems': gastrointestinal and urological. In women a gynaecological cause must also be considered. More unusually it can be a presenting symptom for some systemic illnesses. Possible causes of lower abdominal pain are given in Table 19.1.

Acute appendicitis

Acute appendicitis is usually considered in all cases of lower abdominal pain (see Figure 19.1). Presentation is often classically described as non-specific central abdominal pain (as a result of mid-gut visceral inflammation) that subsequently localises to the right iliac fossa (from parietal peritoneal irritation). Its course is gradual and can present with perforation causing a sudden increase in pain. Sometimes an inflamed appendix causes vague more intermittent pain which can radiate to the right upper quadrant or left iliac fossa, depending on its location and orientation. The patient will often have systemic symptoms such as fever, vomiting and anorexia. Diagnosis is often made clinically with localised tenderness, guarding, rebound and percussion tenderness at McBurney's point

Table 19.1 Causes of lower abdominal pain.

Systems causes	
Gastrointestinal	Acute appendicitis Terminal ileitis • inflammatory • infective Meckel's diverticulitis Colonic pathology • perforation • cancer • diverticulitis Mesenteric • adenitis • ischaemia Pancreatitis (usually generalised)
Urological	Infective • cystitis • pyelonephritis Calculi • renal • ureteric • bladder
Gynaecological	Ovarian • cyst • torsion Infective • salpingitis • endometritis • cervicitis Ectopic pregnancy Endometriosis (cyclical)
Referred	Lower lobe pneumonia Diabetic ketoacidosis Nerve root pain • shingles • spinal lesion

(one-third of the way along line from the anterior superior iliac spine to the umbilicus).

Terminal ileitis

The terminal ileum can become acutely inflamed from both inflammatory and infective causes. Crohn's disease presents before the age of 25 years in about 60% of cases and most

ABC of Emergency Differential Diagnosis. Edited by F. Morris and A. Fletcher.
© 2009 Blackwell Publishing, ISBN: 978-1-4051-7063-5.

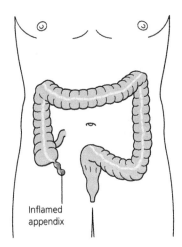

Inflamed
appendix

Figure 19.1 Inflamed appendix.

commonly affects the terminal ileum. On average symptoms are present intermittently for up to 5 years prior to diagnosis. Crohn's disease differs from ulcerative colitis in that it can affect any area of the gastrointestinal tract and involves the whole thickness of the bowel wall (transmural inflammation) leading to serosal inflammation. This can irritate the parietal peritoneum leading to localised pain and tenderness, mimicking appendicitis. There is often a background history of diarrhoea, colicky abdominal pain, weight loss and general malaise (exacerbated during an acute attack) and a careful history may elicit evidence of systemic manifestations of inflammatory bowel disease (see Table 19.2).

Ovarian pain

Ovarian cysts are common and can be considered normal if small (<5 cm). Non-neoplastic cysts are caused by different mechanisms but can cause pain with rupture, haemorrhage or expansion (failure to rupture). Cysts are also found in neoplastic ovarian pathology.

Careful history taking may identify recurrent grumbling pains related to the menstrual cycle and bimanual examination may reveal a palpable ovary or mobile mass. Localised peritonism is a result of the contents of the cyst irritating the peritoneal lining of the abdominal cavity.

A pedunculated cyst or tumour may twist leading to venous occlusion, engorgement and pain that can be intermittent as the torsion twists and untwists. Again a mass would be expected but may not be palpable. Ovarian pathology is usually visible on pelvic ultrasound.

Ovulation pain (mittelschmerz, from the German for middle pain) occurs around day 14 of the menstrual cycle. There is usually a history of previous episodes and it is more common in teenagers and older women.

Pelvic infection (pelvic inflammatory disease)

This is mostly infection of the Fallopian tubes (salpingitis) but can involve other pelvic structures. The most common cause is chlamydial infection from sexual transmission (90%) of cases, with childbirth or instrumentation accounting for 10%. Acute salpingitis presents with fever, severe abdominal pain, nausea

Table 19.2 Systemic manifestations of inflammatory bowel disease.

Anatomical region	Manifestation
Constitutional	Weight loss Malaise Growth retardation Signs of malabsorption
Eyes	Episcleritis Uveitis
Mouth	Aphthous ulcers
Skin	Erythema nodosum Pyoderma gangrenosum
Musculoskeletal (joints)	Entropathic arthropathy • asymmetrical • large joints Sacroiliitis Ankylosing spondylitis Clubbing
Hepatobiliary	Fatty liver Hepatitis • chronic active • granulomatous Cirrhosis Amyloid (rare) Gallstones (terminal ileum disease) Sclerosing cholangitis (UC) Bile-duct carcinoma (UC)
Renal	Ureteric calculi • oxalate (terminal ileum disease) • uric acid (total colitis or ileostomy) Amyloid (rare)
Blood	Anaemia • iron • vitamin B12 • folate Arterial and venous thrombosis

and vomiting and can be localised unilaterally (although is more commonly bilateral pain). There is vaginal discharge with cervicitis and bleeding with endometritis. Vaginal examination will reveal pelvic tenderness and cervical excitation.

Ectopic pregnancy

This occurs in approximately 1 in 100 pregnancies and risk factors include: previous damage to the Fallopian tubes from salpingitis or surgery; previous ectopic pregnancies; endometriosis; IUCD or the progesterone-only pill (see Figure 19.2).

Typical presentation is with sudden onset of lower abdominal pain and vaginal bleeding after a period of amenorrhoea (6–8 weeks). The pain may precede bleeding and radiate to the shoulder tip (suggesting diaphragmatic irritation) or perineum (suggesting pelvic irritation) (see Figure 19.3).

This is a potentially fatal condition and should be considered in all women of childbearing age presenting with acute, severe abdominal pain. Concerning features include localised abdominal peritonism, shock, and history of a collapse.

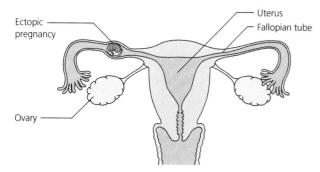

Figure 19.2 Ectopic pregnancy.

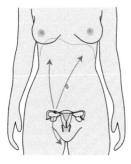

Figure 19.3 Ectopic pregnancy: free blood within the peritoneal cavity can track superiorly to irritate the diaphragm (leading to shoulder tip referred pain), or inferiorly to cause perineal pain.

Renal calculi

There are several causes for calculi including infection, anatomical reasons and hypercalcaemia. Their presentation is dependent on the site of the calculus. Pelvic (staghorn) calculi will present with loin pain and upper urinary tract infection.

Ureteric calculi typically present with severe, colicky unilateral pain radiating from loin to groin and even to testes or labia. They can be associated with haematuria and about 90% are radio-opaque on plain X-ray. It is less common to find abdominal wall tenderness. A common concern is the possibility of an undiagnosed abdominal aortic aneurysm which can present similarly, especially in those over the age of 55 years.

Other causes of lower abdominal pain not suggested by the history

Urinary tract infection

Lower urinary tract infections present with the typical constellation of symptoms of dysuria, frequency, urgency and suprapubic pain. Bedside dipstick testing can guide this diagnosis. Upper tract infections often have associated systemic symptoms of fever, rigors, anorexia with some flank pain and abdominal tenderness.

Caecal cancer

In older people the caecum itself may be abnormal. Caecal distension secondary to large bowel obstruction may cause localised pain and tenderness in the right iliac fossa; however, a palpable mass would usually be present. More generalised abdominal distension is also usually evident but an ascending colon stenosis is possible. Localised caecal malignancy can also lead to peritoneal irritation through local perforation or invasion but again a mass should be palpable.

Meckel's diverticulum

Present in 2% of the population, this remnant of the vitello-intestinal duct forms a blind ending pouch on the terminal ileum, approximately 50 cm from the ileocaecal junction. Mostly asymptomatic this may present with acute or chronic symptoms and can mimic acute appendicitis if inflamed or ruptured. Chronic symptoms include rectal bleeding. A Meckel's diverticulum should always be looked for at operation on finding a normal appendix.

Mesenteric adenitis

More commonly seen in children than adults, inflammation and enlargement of the mesenteric lymph glands can lead to colicky abdominal pain. It is associated with viral illness, often an upper respiratory tract or pharyngeal infection, and may present acutely. Fever is typically higher than with appendicitis (greater than 38.5°C) and resolves rapidly.

Diabetic ketoacidosis

Severe dehydration and ketone production with metabolic acidosis lead to hyperventilation and can cause generalised abdominal pain which can mimic an 'acute abdomen'. It would be unusual to have tenderness in the right iliac fossa.

Case history revisited

Our patient has had grumbling pains for 2 days and presents with sudden, severe pain and collapse. More information is needed from the history for specific conditions to be excluded, for example:
- When was her last period?
- Has she had any fever or rigors?
- Has she had any previous bleeding (per vaginum or per rectum)?
- Have there been any previous abdominal symptoms?

Her recent course of doxycycline is relevant because it was used to treat *Chlamydia* and suggests pelvic infection, but the collapse points towards ectopic pregnancy despite contraception. Ovarian pain, salpingitis, and appendicitis are possibilities because of the site and character of the pain. Urological causes are less likely because of the absence of urinary or colicky symptoms.

Examination

She looks pale and clammy, with cool hands and feet. Observations are: pulse 112 beats/minute, blood pressure 115/85 mmHg, temperature 36.4°C, blood glucose meter 6.7 mmol/l, respiratory rate 30/minute, oxygen saturations 98% on air. Heart and chest examination is normal. There is marked tenderness in the right iliac fossa with peritonism on percussion. The rest of the abdomen is diffusely tender. Urine testing by dipstick reveals no infection but is positive on pregnancy testing.

Question: Given the history and examination findings what is your principal working diagnosis?

Principal working diagnosis – Ruptured ectopic pregnancy

Examination shows cardiovascular compromise with a tachycardia and tachypnoea. Peritonism in the right iliac fossa could represent acute appendicitis and rupture, but the positive pregnancy test makes ectopic pregnancy a principal diagnosis. The normality of the rest of the examination and an otherwise negative urine test makes the rest of the differentials much less likely.

Management

Our patient needs emergency investigation and treatment. She should be resuscitated with oxygen and intravenous fluids via large bore cannulae. Blood tests for urgent cross match, full blood count, and β-HCG should be taken at the same time as an emergency referral to a senior gynaecological surgeon. Utilisation of the FAST ultrasound technique may identify free fluid within the peritoneum or recto-vesical pouch and aid rapid diagnosis.

If ectopic pregnancy is excluded, an alternative diagnosis should be sought. Investigation would include abdominal CT scanning, urethral and endocervical swabs, and a period of careful observation. Investigations supporting a diagnosis of appendicitis include an elevated white cell count (aids in exclusion of non-suppurative gynaecological pathology), negative urinary dipstick (excluding urinary tract infection) and a negative pregnancy test (excluding ectopic pregnancy). None of these investigations can accurately confirm appendicitis, however.

Outcome

Our patient responded to fluid resuscitation and was taken urgently to the operating theatre where a bleeding ectopic pregnancy was ligated and removed. Although she needed a 10 unit blood transfusion perioperatively she made a good recovery. A review of the British National Formulary found doxycycline to be enzyme-inducing, resulting in reduced contraceptive efficacy.

Further reading

Grace PA, Borley NR. *Surgery at a Glance*, Second Edition. Blackwell Publishing, Oxford, 2002.

Moore KL, Dalley AF. *Clinically Oriented Anatomy*, Fourth Edition. Lippincott, Williams & Wilkins, Baltimore, 1999.

Index